The QOD Diet

Eating Well Every Other Day

Set free the REAL you!

- Learn how to fool your body to keep it from switching into starvation mode.
- Use the kidneys' "salt secret" to markedly reduce food intake without feeling woozy or washed out.
- Avoid problems linked to protein-rich ultra-low carb diets.
- Learn to identify your body's specific food hungers.
- Enjoy the mental and spiritual benefits of periodic, comfortable, fasting.

Published by:
White Swan Publishing, Ltd.
15W560 89th Street
Willowbrook, IL 60527

Library of Congress Control Number· 200592`

ISBN-10: 0-9774614-0-8
ISBN-13: 978-097746140-0

Acknowledgment:
The author gratefully acknowledges the help of Ken McFarland, a gifted writer, for his help in putting together the original draft. Many thanks, also, to sons Kestutis and Adomas, for their help in editing and photography. Also, thanks to 1106 Design (*1106design.com*) for cover design and book layout.

Publisher's Cataloging-in-Publication
(Provided by Quality Books, Inc.)

    Daugirdas, John T.
       The QOD diet : eating well every other day / John
    Daugirdas.
       p. cm.
       Includes bibliographical references.
       ISBN 0-9774614-0-8
       1. Reducing diets. 2. Metabolism.   I. Title.
    RM222.2.D299 2006   613.2'5
               QBI05-600186

FOREWORD

Why a diet book from a kidney doctor? We're in the middle of a worldwide epidemic of obesity. Obesity can lead to diabetes, and diabetes can cause heart and kidney damage. Is dieting the solution? It is difficult to diet successfully. If the body is deprived of food for several days, survival and starvation mechanisms kick in and fuel is burned more efficiently. Basically, the body learns to get by with less. So weight is lost at first, but then weight loss ceases, and ultimately, most dieters gain their weight back soon after resuming normal eating.

In the QOD diet, Dr. John Daugirdas—a kidney doctor—has applied his knowledge of physician "tricks" to develop a new kind of diet based on eating mostly every other day that tries to get around this problem of activating starvation mode. What sort of "trick" is used? Physicians, including kidney doctors, sometimes need to suppress the immune system with steroids in order to treat diseases where the immune system has turned against the body. When steroids are given every day, they shut down production of the body's normal stress hormones, causing a variety of side effects. One physician "trick" is to give the steroids *every other day*. This allows the body to rest and recover from the steroid treatments. With an every other day treatment schedule, steroid side effects are minimized.

Daugirdas adapts this physician "trick" to energy metabolism, in order to fool the body into not activating its survival-starvation mode. In his QOD diet, you diet for only a single day at a time—every other day—and these 1-day periods of reduced food intake are not long enough to activate the body's starvation response. The body's thermostat is not turned down so much or so quickly. As long as your average daily intake of calories remains below the body's setpoint, you lose weight.

The question remains—Why a diet book by a *kidney* doctor? The kidneys control the amount of minerals, including salt, in our bodies. If we have too much salt, the kidneys get rid of it. If we have too little salt, the kidneys try to conserve it. Here comes the "salt secret"—what a kidney doctor knows, but others may not: We eat much more salt than we were designed . . . . Most of us adapt to this quite well, and our kidneys pass the excess salt out in urine.

When people fast, they stop eating calories but they also stop taking in minerals, including salt. It takes the kidney several days to cut back from its "Let's get rid of all this extra salt" mode. Plus, fasting by itself, by causing ketosis, makes the kidneys excrete more salt and water in the urine. So for the first day or two of fasting, a lot of salt and water continue to be lost in the urine, more than is good for the body. This loss of salt and water can lower the blood volume, and as a result, a person can feel weak and woozy. They think "I just can't be without food for even half a day. I feel so washed out!"

So the "salt secret" is to keep up your intake of minerals, especially sodium, during fasting to prevent salt loss by the kidneys and volume depletion. This makes the every other day diet easy to tolerate. Also, the QOD fast is only a partial fast—some carbs and other foods are taken in. A mild fast limits the tendency of the kidneys to lose so much salt and water.

Kidney doctors also know that you lose calcium in the urine every day, whether you eat or not, and that potassium and magnesium are good for you. So the QOD diet recommends a continuing, daily intake of calcium, potassium, and magnesium, even while dieting every other day.

Kidney doctors know, too, that very low carbohydrate diets have a dark side. When the body metabolizes most proteins, a little bit of acid is left behind. The kidneys normally put this acid out in the urine. But the more protein you take in, the more acid you put into your kidneys. The kidneys can get rid of this, but in doing so, you lose large amounts of calcium in the urine. A little bit of extra calcium lost in the urine each day, and you can wind up with osteoporosis in your old age. The high amount of meat taken in with low-carbohydrate diets may be bad for you as well. Most meats and many other protein-rich foods contain large amounts of purines, which are building blocks of DNA. Purines are broken down by the body into uric acid, and high levels of uric acid can lead to kidney stones, and there are new theories suggesting that high uric-acid levels can contrib   rtension and cardiovascular disease[1].

The QOD diet allows people to eat a healthful balance of proteins, fats and good carbs. It's a way of dieting that can help people avoid being caught in the current epidemic of obesity, with all of its serious consequences. It's not for patients with eating disorder tendencies, nor for patients with serious medical problems, nor for those who need to take medications for diabetes, heart disease, hypertension, stroke, or other conditions, but it is a way to help healthy people lose a moderate amount of weight and then to maintain their weight.

CONTENTS

CHAPTER 1

WHAT IS QOD?

T HE QOD DIET concept is simple. There are no long lists of foods to avoid and there is no need to focus on eating primarily one or two classes of food. Instead, the QOD diet alternates ON days when you *eat well* with OFF days, when you restrict food intake and give your body a rest. Although we refer to the OFF days as days of fasting, this is not quite accurate: You do take in a small amount of calories and relatively large amounts of certain key minerals and critical nutrients.

The great thing about the QOD diet is that it's effective in multiple ways. You will lose weight if you have the discipline to follow the plan. And not only will it help you lose weight, you will enjoy additional benefits for your body, mind and spirit.

We'll get into more details later in the book and I've also included recipes, but as an introduction, here's how the QOD diet works:

The OFF days

On your OFF days—those alternating days when you restrict your food intake—you'll be able to eat up to 400 calories. You will need to count your calories carefully. About half of these calories

1

should be from juices that contain lots of sodium and potassium but that don't contain too many calories. Tomato juice or vegetable juice is best. The remaining calories are taken in as small, 25- to 50-calorie "mini-meals" that will provide you with just enough fuel to stay energized.

The ON days

On your ON days, you'll be able to eat pretty much anything you want. As long as you are careful not to binge eat, to limit the size of each meal, and eat only one dessert per day, you will be able to eat as much food as you need to feel satisfied. Even if you eat a bit more than usual, your average food intake will be significantly reduced because of the small amount eaten during the OFF days.

The start of your journey

That's the basic idea. Simple, right? It really is. The QOD diet isn't new. Alternate-day fasting has been around for more than a thousand years in one form or another. Eating QOD not only achieves weight loss, but also may be useful in resting the body and clarifying the mind.

The hard part is developing the discipline it will take to stick with the diet. But that's true of anything that brings long-lasting, positive results. To enjoy the benefits of this simple, effective diet, you'll have to commit yourself and not give up. If you're willing to dedicate yourself to following the QOD guidelines, you *will* achieve results. You *will* lose weight. And, not only will you look and feel better, but you very well may add years to your life.

What's in the name?

QOD is an acronym representing both Latin and English words.

The "Q" is for the Latin word *"quaque,"* which means "every." The "O" is for the English word *"other"* and the "D", well that means "day", or as they say in Latin, *"die"*—***Quaque Other Die***—**Every Other Day.**

CHAPTER 2

QOD IS NOT FOR EVERYONE

W HEN THE FIRST Model T rolled off the assembly line in 1914, it came in just one color: black. Henry Ford had discovered that black paint dried faster than any other color, so his factories could make more cars in less time by painting them black. It wouldn't be until 1926 that cars came in any other color. Today, you can get a car in just about any color imaginable, including, of course, black. The assembly line that Henry Ford pioneered may have worked for cars, but human beings are each custom-made. We have different tastes, preferences, likes, and dislikes. Our personalities, temperaments, attitudes, personal histories, goals, and interests—all of these vary dramatically from one person to another.

And we're also custom-made biologically. The DNA—the genetic code—of each of the 6.5 billion people on Planet Earth is different from that of all others. That means your own personal physiology is not shared by anyone else. Your brain and blood chemistry are unique—as is your metabolism, your responses to food and your sensitivity to drugs.

That's why a drug that will work well for one person may not work so well, or at all, for someone else. This difference between people also means that there is no diet approach that will achieve the same results for everyone who tries it.

> An entire field of research has arisen which studies how a person's genetic inheritance affects the body's responses to drugs. This focus of study is called pharmacogenomics.

And since one size doesn't fit all, even a seemingly effective diet plan may not be right for everyone. There are certain people for whom eating QOD may not be right or advisable. There are certain tendencies or conditions that some people have, that could make this diet approach ineffective or even unsafe.

The QOD diet is meant for basically healthy people who need to lose 25 lbs or less. It may be particularly useful for people who want to tune up their body every once in a while by losing a small amount of weight. It is not designed for people who are massively obese nor for people with serious health problems. The QOD diet is not designed to treat any chronic disease. Also, the QOD diet is designed for young and middle-aged adults. **It is not meant for children nor for people over 60 years of age.** If you are under a doctor's care, before you consider going on a QOD eating plan, always check with him or her first.

In addition to the above, people for whom the QOD diet may not be appropriate include:

Those with a tendency toward binge eating or other eating disorders[1]

Eating QOD consists of alternating ON and OFF days—a cyclical pattern which may parallel too closely the alternating pattern of those who binge eat and then purge, or who binge eat even without purging. While the ON and OFF pattern of QOD will not pose a

> There is no diet approach that will achieve the same results for everyone. And even the most effective diet plans may not be right for everyone.

problem to the majority of people, that may not be true for those who struggle with eating disorders such as anorexia or binge eating syndromes. Eating very large amounts of food, especially quickly, is never healthy and may be dangerous. By the same token, if you have ever suffered from anorexia—which is basically defined as starving yourself to the point that you become malnourished—going on a cyclical diet like QOD may make this worse.

If you have a tendency to binge eat or have ever had anorexia, *you should not* attempt the QOD way of eating.

Those who have either had a heart attack or are at increased risk for a heart attack[2]

There is some recent evidence that the risk of a heart attack may be markedly increased after eating a large meal, and in particular, a large, fatty meal. If you are following the QOD diet properly, you should be eating multiple, moderate sized meals and avoiding large meals during the ON day—but some might be tempted to eat this way during the ON day. The QOD diet is not for you.

Those who are diabetic

Diabetic medications have been designed for people eating three meals per day. With some medications, like insulin, the amount of insulin given is linked closely to the estimated amount of carbohydrates being taken in. With the QOD approach, significantly fewer calories and carbs are consumed over the course of the OFF days and this can throw off the balance between medications and carbohydrate intake. Also, some diabetic patients don't tolerate fasting well. For this reason, QOD is not advisable for anyone taking diabetes medications.

Those who need to restrict or monitor their sodium or potassium intake for any reason

Some people, for health reasons, need to be following a low-sodium diet. While the sodium intake recommended in the QOD diet is not high, it may be higher than that recommended for you.

Potassium is a mineral that's good for you. Most of us don't get enough. However, some people with kidney disease or on certain medications have to restrict how much potassium-containing foods they eat because their kidneys have trouble excreting potassium. Some commonly used medications impair the ability of the kidneys to excrete potassium. So if you are taking any kind of medication that affects potassium (most often ACE inhibitors, aldosterone blockers, or certain antibiotics) or if you have impaired kidney function, the QOD diet, which focuses on eating potassium-rich foods, is not for you unless you follow this diet while under close supervision of your doctor.

Those with high blood pressure or with heart or kidney disease, and especially those taking water pills

Another group of people for whom QOD could be problematic are those receiving medical treatment for high blood pressure or heart or kidney disease. Some blood pressure and heart medications—just like some diabetes medications—are designed with certain expectations. It's assumed that a patient being treated for hypertension, for example, will maintain a relatively constant level of sodium intake every day. This is particularly true of the class of blood pressure medications called *diuretics*—which are designed to remove excess salt and water from the tissues. During the OFF days you will tend to lose sodium and water, and it may be difficult for your physician to adjust these medications appropriately. If you have high blood pressure, heart disease or have had a stroke and you still want to follow the QOD diet, your sodium intake, potassium intake (see above) and medications must be carefully monitored by your doctor.

Those with low blood pressure, dizziness, or history of fainting, stroke or near-stroke[3]

Food intake can make your blood pressure fall. Why? More blood is shifted to your intestines. So the heart has to pump more blood, and because more blood is going to the intestines, if you're a bit dried out, or if your blood vessels aren't able to adjust properly, blood pressure can fall. This sort of thing is worse especially after a large meal containing lots of carbs. Elderly people sometimes get dizzy after a meal, especially after standing up, and especially if they are taking water pills. This is because their blood vessels can't adjust as well as those in younger people. Diabetics have this problem sometime because of nervous system damage due to diabetes. For this reason I don't recommend QOD eating for people over 60, and also don't recommend for anyone who has suffered from dizziness, low blood pressure, or any sort of problems related to stroke. Again, when eating QOD, I recommend eating 5–6 small meals per day, but for added safety, if you have such problems, the QOD diet is not for you.

Those taking long-term prescription medications, absorption of which is affected by food intake[4]

Food intake can affect the absorption of many types of drugs. Usually absorption is reduced on a full stomach. Absorption of such drugs might be different during days when caloric intake is high (ON days) vs. when it is low (OFF days), giving you ups and downs in terms of drug effect. If you are being treated with prescription medication for any condition, always consult with your doctor before going on the QOD diet.

QOD may be difficult for those who don't like vegetables, and especially, tomatoes, and/or tomato juice

The QOD eating plan relies on eating potassium-rich, low calorie vegetables, and particularly, makes use of tomato juice and vegetable juices containing tomato juice. Vegetables are one of the few ways you can eat a restricted amount of calories and yet get a good supply of potassium. You can probably work out a system of eating QOD without tomato juice, and we have some suggestions in this area, but the eating plan is much easier if you are able to drink tomato-containing vegetable juice on a regular basis.

For the rest, QOD will help you win at losing

Now, it's possible that others besides those we've specifically mentioned here will attempt the QOD approach and find that it simply is not a good fit for them. But I'm confident that most people will find QOD effective, physically invigorating and mentally clarifying. They will not only tolerate well the QOD eating pattern, but will find themselves happily winning at losing!

Do I qualify for eating QOD?

1. I am basically healthy
2. I am less than 25 lbs overweight
3. I am 20–60 years of age
4. I don't mind eating tomatoes and other vegetables
5. I have no tendency to binge eating or anorexia
6. I have no heart disease
7. I am not a diabetic
8. I have no kidney disease or hypertension
9. I have no history of low blood pressure, dizziness, fainting, or stroke or near-stroke
10. I have no reason to restrict sodium or potassium
11. I am not taking medications that interact with food or potassium
12. I am not taking any type of water pills (diuretics)

For more detailed information see comments in Appendix A.

CHAPTER 3

WHY EATING EVERY OTHER DAY DOES WORK
(AND WHY MANY DIETS FAIL)

T he rate of obesity is rising at an alarming rate in the United States; some say, to epidemic proportions. Why is this happening? People are eating more and exercising less. Why eating more? Supersized portions, soft drinks, food available everywhere. Why exercising less? Computers, video games, television.

Your Body's "Red Alert" Response

If eating can lead to weight gain, when you eat less, shouldn't you automatically lose weight? What if we just fasted totally until we got down to the weight we'd like to be? Wouldn't that be the quickest way to reach our goal?

Well, yes and no. To understand this better, you need to understand some basic concepts about *metabolism.* Metabolism is similar

Obesity is associated with many serious medical conditions. A study reported in the *Journal of the American Medical Association* showed that obesity was associated with at least 110,000 excess deaths per year in the United States.[1]

to the engine in your car that converts fuel into energy. Instead of gasoline, you burn food for fuel. Food contains *potential* energy in the form of **calories**.

When your body metabolizes the food you eat, the *potential* energy contained within food (measured as calories) is released as *kinetic* energy—the kind that moves your arms and legs and makes you active, plus other forms of energy needed to maintain various bodily functions.

Some people metabolize food (burn fuel) more or less efficiently than do others. Also, the rate at which you burn food for energy can be influenced by many things: weight, age, sex, genetic factors, activity levels, even thyroid gland function.

The most important point is that the rate of metabolism is also affected by how much food we eat. Our bodies have evolved to help keep us alive during periods of both feast and famine. When you significantly reduce your food intake for more than a few days, your body becomes your enemy, simply by doing the job that it has been programmed to do. Your body interprets the lower food intake as the beginning of starvation—a threat to survival—and takes measures to defend itself. It doesn't know that you only plan to cut back temporarily until you reach your ideal weight. So your body goes into survival mode by slowing down the rate at which you burn food for energy—it reduces your metabolism to conserve both your energy output and your potentially life-saving stores of fat.

Because of this starvation response, on almost any diet you'll lose a few pounds quickly—mostly excess water. But before long, you find it harder and harder to continue losing weight, even though you are eating far less than you used to eat. In time, you may find yourself stuck on a weight-loss "plateau," unable to lose more, even while eating less.

One (kilo)calorie is equal to the amount of heat needed to raise the temperature of one liter of water by one degree Celsius.

In such situations, psychologically, it's hard to endure ongoing feelings of hunger or deprivation when there's not much to show for it. So all too often, you abandon the diet and return to eating as you did before. Only now, your body has lowered its metabolism to a much lower point—and you rapidly regain most or all of the pounds that were lost. Sometimes, you gain even more weight so that you wind up heavier than when you started!

Talk about a no-win situation!

The QOD Solution

QOD solves the problem of having to fight against the body's internal survival programming by not triggering "red alert." You see, it takes a few days for the body to "notice" that it isn't getting its regular quota of fuel in the form of food. So when you sneak in a quick fast lasting only a day (your OFF day), you get all the benefit of reducing calories, but you don't cut off the fuel long enough for the alarms to go off, or to send your body into defensive mode.

QOD requires discipline and determination, but because it works in harmony with your body—not against it—it will bring you results. And those results won't just be seen on the scale. Your body, mind and spirit will all benefit from following the QOD diet.

> For those who are science buffs, a recent paper by Leonie Heilbronn and colleagues from Baton Rouge, LA, put 8 men and 8 women on a QOD-style diet—an alternate day fast—for 22 days. This was a strict fast, with no carbs, calories or mineral intake on the OFF days (ouch!). The subjects' metabolic rates were measured at the outset and 22 days later. After 22 days, there was no significant fall in metabolic rate.[2]

CHAPTER 4

THE KEYS TO QOD SUCCESS
SOLID BASE, BALANCE AND MODERATION

W E ALL KNOW that a solid foundation is critical to a well-built house. According to the Biblical parable[1] (slightly modified for effect), there once were two men. Each wanted to build a house for himself and his family. One summer day, in a pleasant valley, they were both out looking for building sites. One man decided to build on sandy soil where the costs to build would be less and where it would be easier to dig a foundation. The other man decided to build up on a rock. He knew it would cost more and take longer, but he was sure it was a safer place to build.

The two men started building at the same time. The house on the valley floor was finished well ahead of the other home, but eventually the house on the hill was completed as well. Both families moved into their new residences and were quite happy for a time. Then one night there was a huge thunderstorm with pouring rain. The house in the valley was carried away with its inhabitants while the house on the bluff was unharmed.

The moral of the story is this: Anything we ever do in life goes better when we make sure we've got a solid foundation underneath us. What's true of building a house is just as true of rebuilding one's body through changes in diet and exercise. So, before we get into the specifics of reshaping your body's "house" by eating QOD, here are a few suggestions that should increase your chances of success while dieting.

1.   Stock healthy foods in your home

Unless you go to a restaurant or take　　　　　can eat only what you have available in your refrigerator and pantry. If these contain primarily ice cream and cookies, you will wind up eating more carbs and saturated fats and trans-saturated fatty acids than is healthy for you.

Instead, keep a variety of healthy foods in your refrigerator, especially fruits, vegetables, nuts, and healthy oils, so that you will have a variety of good alternatives to choose from. Also, with rare exceptions, don't keep carbohydrate-rich, salty or sugary snacks in your home, such as cookies, chips and ice cream—at least not while you are trying to lose weight or if you are having trouble maintaining your desired weight.

2.   Eat a good balance of fats, proteins and carbohydrates

The hallmark of far too many diet fads is emphasizing one of the three primary components of our food—fats, proteins and carbohydrates—at the expense of another. For years, ultra-low-fat diets were the rage. The food industry jumped onto this bandwagon and cranked out low-fat versions of just about every food product imaginable—even desserts and dairy products. Then the pendulum swung again, and low-carb diets became fashionable. However, these

---

If you like guidelines, you can look at the Dietary Guidelines for Americans, published by the US Dept. of Agriculture, Jan 12, 2005; web address:[2] *health.gov/dietaryguidelines/.*

If you want to know about specific foods, please look at Appendix A in this report: *health.gov/dietaryguidelines/dga2005/document/html/appendixA.htm* and this lists the types of grains, vegetables, fruits, dairy, meats, nut-seed-oil food group, and fats and oils you should be eating in order to take in the nutrients that you need.

can lead one to eat too much protein and fat. The truth is, that we need all three classes of food in a sensible ratio. Too much of any one category creates its own unique health problems. Too much protein can create far too much acid, leach calcium, and stress the kidneys. Too much fat—particularly the wrong kinds of fat—can leave us lacking in many of the vitamins, minerals, and other nutrients found in carbohydrates and proteins, and eating too much saturated fat can lead to heart and blood vessel disease. Cutting out all fat is a bad idea as well. We *need* **unsaturated** fats in our diet in order to remain healthy. Beneficial fats include the omega fats found in oily fish, flaxseed and walnuts. Also, there may be beneficial substances in saturated fats—we just need to eat them in moderation. Eating too many carbohydrates—particularly the highly refined, sugary kind—also is not good. An excess of rapidly digestible carbs upsets the delicate balance of insulin, metabolism and blood glucose levels. This is why eating lots of sugary sweets can lead to carb craving and an appetite without end.

3. Avoid soft drinks. Instead drink flavored water

Americans drink far too many soft drinks, to the great detriment of their health and weight. The average American consumes more than a can-and-a-half of soda pop every day. Soft drinks are the *single biggest source of refined sugar* for Americans, providing the average person with one-third of their daily sugar consumption; even more in 12- to 19-year-old boys and girls.[3]

So please avoid sugary soft drinks altogether (and this includes iced tea and lemonade made from powdered mixes, which are almost pure sugar!). Instead, keep bottles of water handy. For flavor, add a quarter teaspoonful of your favorite jam, or a splash of orange juice, to a large glass of water. If you need some sweet taste, add a teaspoonful of Splenda™ (sucralose). Similarly, when you go to a restaurant or a fast-food place, always ask for water—never for pop or soda. You will save both money and your health.

You might think that it's OK to drink diet soft drinks. I don't recommend it. Research has shown that people who drink a lot of diet drinks actually tend to become obese, probably because the body gets used to eating sweet foods. You need to train your body to be happy with a bit less sweet taste, especially in terms of what you drink. For the same reason, you should be careful in how much low-calorie sweetener you add to your water and other drinks.

4. Watch your portion sizes and avoid binge eating

We've all seen the "supersizing" of ⸱ ⸱ ⸱ ⸱ ⸱s in this country. Many fast-food outlets offer mammoth meals. Plate and portion sizes at restaurants have steadily grown for several decades, and supermarkets offer foods in ever larger containers.

It's wrong. Our bodies were not meant to consume such large quantities. Eating huge portions means you are overeating. You are taking in more fuel than you need. And what happens to fuel that isn't needed immediately? It's stored—in *fat* cells. Also, eating large meals at one sitting, especially those that contain a lot of saturated fat, may actually be dangerous to your health—there is some evidence that blood clots and even heart attacks can occur after a very large, fatty meal.

Do not buy into the all-you-can-eat mentality. Do not follow the herd. To be successful at losing or even maintaining weight, you must control portion sizes. For the most part, it's not what we eat that causes weight gain—it's *how much*. Even the most nutritious foods, eaten in excessive quantities, will lead to an expanding waistline.

One problem is regularly dining out in all-you-can-eat buffet-style restaurants, where you can load up and eat as much food as you want. These restaurants are a good deal, but if you go to them, put in half as much of each food as you would otherwise, then eat it slowly, and think twice before going back for more. My father used to tell me: "When you finish eating, you should be able to sit down and still eat the same amount of food a second time. Otherwise, you've eaten too much." It's good advice.

Another word of caution. One very serious problem, especially among teenagers, is binge eating. Binge eaters consume an inordinate amount of food at one sitting or in the course of one day. This also is called bulimia. Sometimes this is combined with self-induced vomiting (purging). Research shows that going on almost any kind of diet can increase binge eating behavior as people start focusing more on food and hunger. If you find yourself starting to binge eat, stop dieting right away.

The message is simple: Don't stuff yourself. Eat in moderation.

5. Keep an eye on your sodium intake

Research suggests a link between high sodium intake and hypertension for a substantial percentage of people such as the elderly, African Americans and people with impaired kidney function. Many people from these groups have trouble excreting excess salt. Also, for pretty much everyone, a high sodium intake can result in increased loss of calcium in the urine, which over the long term can lead to osteoporosis. For all of these reasons, it is prudent to watch your sodium intake.

So how much sodium is too much? The recommended upper limit for sodium intake for Caucasians in the United States is 2300 milligrams (2.3 grams) per day. An upper limit of 1500 milligrams is recommended for African Americans, for people with high blood pressure and for middle-aged and older adults.[2] Despite these recommendations, the majority of Americans usually take in considerably more sodium than this each day.

You may suspect that foods that taste salty, such as potato chips, are high in total sodium content. But what many may not realize is that many prepared or processed foods are even higher in sodium content. Sauces, soups, chilies, sausages, pizza—even when consumed in

---

More information

For more information on recommended daily sodium levels, see the Dietary Guidelines for Americans, US Dept. of Agriculture:[2] *health.gov/dietaryguidelines/*.

Company websites

Check out the websites of fast-food restaurants to find out exactly what's in the food they serve, including sodium levels.

average portion sizes—can contribute close to an entire daily sodium recommendation. A single bagel can have well over 500 milligrams (mg) of sodium in it—that's more than in some bags of potato chips! Some bread, especially French bread, also contains a lot of salt, even though it doesn't taste salty.

Not only are many common supermarket items loaded with sodium, so also is much of the food served in fast-food or sit-down restaurants. You might be surprised by the levels in that box of fried chicken or plate of spaghetti. If interested you can usually go to fast-food company websites and get nutritional information.

One other often unsuspected source of dietary sodium is softened water, in which sodium is added to the water as part of the softening process. If you consume softened water, consider buying bottled water to drink to reduce your sodium intake.

There's something else you can do to cut back on your sodium intake besides reading food labels: stop adding salt to food during cooking. Many Americans routinely add salt to just about everything as they cook. Into the saucepan with the water and pasta goes what? Salt. The ubiquitous ingredient in nearly any recipe? Salt.

Stop doing that. Instead, use salt only from the shaker. Sprinkle a bit of salt on the surface of your food rather than saturating your food with it during cooking. You will wind up taking in less sodium.

You also will make a rather amazing discovery as you cut back on sodium. At first, your food may taste unpleasantly bland. But before long, your taste buds will adjust to the reduced sodium so

---

The terms *sodium* and *salt* often are used interchangeably. But without getting too technical, they are not the same. Salt is sodium chloride. About 40% by weight of table salt is sodium. On food labels, salt content is listed as sodium, in milligrams (mg). You can easily be fooled, though, by portion sizes. The question to ask is: How much sodium PER CALORIE of food does this item contain? Foods that contain 1 mg sodium per calorie or more are relatively high in sodium (since other foods you eat contain almost no sodium). Pizza, chips, and high-sodium bread contain 2 mg sodium per calorie. Canned soups and chili can sometimes contain 5 mg sodium or more per calorie! Processed foods account for almost 80% of the sodium that we eat.

well that, were you to suddenly return to your old levels of sodium intake, it might feel as if your mouth was burning.

In addition, after those first few initial days during which food tasted relatively bland, something unexpected happens. From those same foods that had seemed to have little taste, new flavor begins to emerge—sometimes distinctive, sometimes subtle, but never noticed until now.

Limit. , sodium intake. is advisable if you plan to shed pounds by following the QOD diet. Spend a few days reducing your sodium intake before you begin Day One of QOD.

6. Make sure you get adequate daily amounts of key nutrients

Certain vitamins, minerals, and other nutrients are readily available in the foods we eat. But not everything we need is easily obtained in this way. Some minerals and vitamins need to be added to our diets in order to reach levels that provide optimum benefits.

Potassium

Whereas a high sodium intake is not good for you, a high potassium intake has been shown to associate with a lower risk of stroke, cardiovascular disease and blood vessel damage. The current recommendation for potassium intake by the US Department of Agriculture is 4700 mg per day.[2] Again, as for sodium, this is a target and does not reflect reality. Actual daily potassium intake in adults in the United States is considerably lower. Why so low? We are not eating our fruits and vegetables!

A diet developed by the National Heart, Lung, and Blood Institute specifically to help decrease blood pressure—the DASH Diet[4]—emphasizes eating fruits and vegetables, and so has higher levels of potassium. Good sources of potassium include:

Vegetables: Tomatoes, broccoli, peas, lima beans, potatoes, leafy green vegetables

Fruits: Citrus, apples, bananas, apricots (especially dried apricots)

Fish: Salmon, cod, flounder, sardines

You can also find out more about foods high in potassium in Appendix B of the USDA Dietary Guidelines for America:[2] *health.gov/dietaryguidelines/dga2005/document/html/appendixB.htm*

Magnesium

Magnesium is another mineral that's important. Deficiencies have been associated with car...ar disease and bone disease. Magnesium is found in many of the same foods that are high in potassium. If you make sure that you eat fruits and vegetables that contain enough potassium, the magnesium will take care of itself.

Calcium

We know that most Americans eat far too much sodium. When we excrete all that excess sodium, some extra calcium is lost in the urine. Over time, a calcium deficiency can occur, which can lead to osteoporosis. Official guidelines recommend an average daily calcium intake for adults of 1000–1300 mg per day, depending on gender and age. See: *iom.edu/Object.File/Master/21/372/0.pdf.*[2]

To take in sufficient calcium to meet guidelines, most people will need to eat a lot of milk products, since milk is one food that has a lot of calcium in it. (Certain vegetables, like broccoli, as well as sardines, also have a lot of calcium.) One problem with milk is that many people (almost all African Americans and Hispanics) can't digest lactose, a sugar that's in milk. They get gas, indigestion, and an upset stomach whenever they try to drink milk. Such people are said to have *lactose intolerance.* My own favorite food is a drinkable yogurt that goes under several different names—in our area it's called Kefir or Kwashenka. In yogurt, most of the lactose has been digested away by the bacteria that turns milk into yogurt. Because of this, many people with lactose-intolerance can digest yogurt without too many problems. Cheese is an alternative source of calcium but most cheese contains a lot of saturated fat. Some dairy products, by the way, such as cottage cheese and sour cream, contain relatively little calcium (but lots of fat).

Calcium is now being added to many foods such as orange juice and breads and breakfast cereals. Of these, orange juice is one source that I particularly recommend, because it's an excellent source of potassium as well.

Vitamin D

The best way to get enough vitamin D is to spend time outdoors in the sunshine—which is the ultimate source of this necessary vitamin. Unfortunately, many people hardly ever stay outdoors. Even in sunny areas, people move from house to car (with tinted windows) to office and back again, minimizing their exposure to the sun. In northern latitudes, where the amount of sunshine is limited, both children and adults rarely get enough vitamin D from the sun.

In earlier centuries, a vitamin D deficiency would result in a soft-bone disease called rickets. While rickets is no longer a health problem, vitamin D is still necessary for optimal health. Research shows that vitamin D has beneficial effects for the immune system and might also help protect against certain forms of cancer.

From dietary sources, your daily multivitamin, and possibly a vitamin D supplement, you should be getting at least 800 IU (international units) of vitamin D per day. Usually a multivitamin will contain about 400 units of vitamin D. You also can buy vitamin pills that contain only vitamin D, usually 400 IU per tablet.

The B Vitamins and Vitamin C

All of the B vitamins are important to good health, but three that I would like to specifically recommend to you are pyridoxine, folic acid, and vitamin B-12 (known also as cobalamin).

Insufficiency of folic acid and/or B-12 is linked to anemia, fatigue, and nervous system disorders. Pyridoxine is essential to many vital body processes, including the production of hemoglobin and the metabolizing of protein. Folic acid is needed to protect against fetal malformations. More importantly, recent evidence suggests that folic acid, pyridoxine, and B-12 are all involved in maintaining the health of the cardiovascular system. Together the   ody to metabolize an amino acid called homocysteine. High blood homocysteine levels have been associated with an increased risk of heart and blood vessel disease, so keeping levels low is beneficial to your health.

A good super-B-complex supplement will protect against reduced intake of folate and pyridoxine and ensure that you don't have a chronic deficiency. Vitamin B-12 is another story. Vitamin B-12 supplementation is particularly important for vegetarians or vegans, as B-12 is found almost exclusively in animal sources. Others who need to take special care to get enough B-12 are older people. The stomach secretes *intrinsic factor* to help absorb vitamin B-12. With aging, the glands of the stomach can atrophy, and vitamin B-12 absorption may become reduced. The minimum daily requirement of B-12, currently 2.5 micrograms/day, is much too low if you need to correct a deficiency. Research suggests that vitamin B-12 deficiency is not uncommon in elderly patients, and that 300–1000 micrograms of oral vitamin B-12 per day is required for correction.[5] The good news is, usually you don't need vitamin B-12 shots as in the past.

Vitamin C, the vitamin that is used to prevent scurvy, is another very important vitamin. The trend these days is to take no more than about 300 mg/day of vitamin C. The minimum daily requirement is 60 mg/day.

7. Fiber and Water

Fiber is important. If you don't eat enough fiber you will become constipated. Plus, fiber is good for you; a diet high in fiber has been linked to a reduced risk of cancer and heart disease and to lower blood levels of cholesterol. The experts recommend about 38 g intake per day in men and 25 or so grams in women[2] (most people eat considerably less). It's hard to get enough fiber unless you eat unrefined grain bread and lots of fruits and vegetables. When limiting food intake during dieting, a fiber supplement is usually necessary.

Water is another important element to any diet. Sometimes people mistake hunger for thirst, so keeping your water intake high may help limit your food intake. Also, if you don't drink enough water or other fluids, you may become constipated.

8. Find Your Golden Mean

Aristotle and Confucius were philosophers, not dietitians. But some of what they taught certainly applies whenever you and I sit down to eat. Both philosophers believed in something that has come to be known as the "Golden Mean" between opposite extremes.[6]

They taught that any virtue can be found between the extremes of excess or deficiency. Likewise, any virtue taken to an extreme can become a vice. For example, courage is a virtue. But taken to an extreme of deficiency, courage becomes the vice of cowardice. Taken to an extreme of excess, courage becomes the vice of recklessness.

What the philosophers taught also holds true for eating. Taken to the extreme of excess, eating becomes the vice of gluttony. Taken to the extreme of deficiency, it becomes the vice of starvation and anorexia.

The "Golden Mean" applies not just to how much or how little we eat. It also applies to what we eat, when and even how. The whole idea, when it comes to our eating, is to find that golden mean of *balance*. Another good word to describe that middle ground would be *moderation*.

Measured by that yardstick, much of today's dietary advice comes up short. Faced with a constantly changing variety of diet and weight-loss plans, it's no wonder that those who want to lose weight often feel overwhelmed. Many have tried one diet after another without lasting success, yet they keep hoping to finally find one that works.

I line up with Confucius and Aristotle. I believe wholeheartedly in avoiding extremes and striving for balance and moderation. Lasting weight loss and better health are found in the middle.

CHAPTER 5

THE OFF DAY: USING THE "SALT SECRET" TO KEEP UP YOUR ENERGY LEVEL

You'll be moving and learning!

You're about to embark on an adventure. You will be moving from a "fed" to a "fasted" state. For many of you, the feeling will be something you've never experienced, or have long forgotten. Primitive man appears to have been designed to operate mostly in a "fasting" state. Long periods of fasting would be interspersed with times when man would succeed at the hunt and eat his fill, thus entering a "fed" state.

Today, however—at least in developed countries of the world, and most certainly in America—people virtually never enter the "fasting" state. A whole world of powerful factors—upbringing, advertising enticements, easy availability, social conventions and just personal habit—push Americans to constantly stay in the "fed" state.

People often eat for a variety of emotional reasons. Many fall into the pattern of eating when anxious, depressed, fearful or bored. They eat for comfort and solace, or as a form of emotional anesthesia. This constant eating can for many become an almost mindless activity. It's so easy to sit in front of a TV and snack, munch and graze for hours, with not a thought as to how many calories one is taking in. And what would a day at the ballpark be without hotdogs and sugar-laden sodas? What would an outing to the movies be without popcorn saturated in butter, a box of candy and soft drinks, plus a trip to the local fast-food outlet afterward?

As a result of all this eating—this constant living within the "fed" state—people end up with carb cravings bordering on addiction. They develop insulin imbalances that ~~~~~~~~~ body to store fat. They also end up eating far too much dietary fat—far too many calories—far too many carbs.

By deliberately choosing to get out of the "fed" state and experience the "fasting" state, you will gain many valuable benefits. Choosing to eat every other day, you'll finally be able to break the cycle of emotional, scheduled, or habitual eating. You'll get away from constant eating even when you're not hungry. At long last, you'll give your body a chance to "talk" to you during a time of rest—you'll learn how to "listen" to what it says to you. You'll learn to distinguish between real hunger and mindless, "automatic" eating that has little to do with genuine hunger. You'll quiet your longstanding cravings and find that you can trust your body to "tell" you which foods it *really* needs.

Five basic principles for OFF day eating

So if you are committed to try QOD eating, let's get started! The QOD diet is simple: OFF day, ON day, OFF day, ON day. You can begin with the OFF day. How much food should you eat? What types of food? When should you eat? There are five guiding principles or food goals for the OFF days:

1) **1500–2000[1] mg sodium/2000 mg potassium:** Through your food, you want to take in 1500–2000 mg of sodium and 2000 mg of potassium.

2) **1000 mL (32 oz) water:** You need to take in *at least* 32 oz of water (1000 mL) in addition to the juices and other liquids that you drink.

3) **300–400 calories:** You can eat food, but only 300–400 calories worth. Food should be eaten throughout the day. About half of your calories will come from 3 nutritionally rich juices, and the rest from 25- to 50-calorie vegetable or fruit mini-meals, taken throughout the day.

4) **Eat at least 20 g of high-biologic-value protein** (dairy, soy).

5) **Fiber, calcium, and vitamins:** You will need to take supplements: fiber, calcium, and vitamin D. Other vitamins (B and C) are optional.

Principle 1: Take in 1500–2000[1] mg of sodium and 2000 mg of potassium

Sodium

Many people find fasting—even for half a day—to be nearly impossible. They begin to feel dizzy and weak. When this happens, it's easy for some to conclude that their blood sugar is low and that therefore they need to eat—when in fact, their blood sugar may not be low at all. The body has compensatory mechanisms that keep the level of sugar in the blood up during a fast. I believe that complete cessation of salt intake—such as during a fast—is what leaves most people feeling very weak and washed out.

If you're like most people, you take in a lot of salt each day. Your kidneys have adjusted to this higher salt level, and have "programmed" themselves to excrete the salt (sodium) your body doesn't need through urination. When you fast, it normally takes your kidneys a couple of days to adjust to the lower salt intake, so on the first day of a fast—such as your OFF day—your kidneys continue to excrete a large amount of sodium. If you don't take in enough sodium on your OFF day, the sodium content of your body falls and along with it, the amount of water. There is a second issue. During fasting, your body begins to switch its metabolism and goes into what is known as *ketosis*. While ketosis is a good thing because it cuts down on your appetite, it can cause problems because it increases loss of sodium and water in the urine.

So without enough salt, the volume of water in your body, as well as of the blood circulating in your body can begin to fall. This lowered blood volume can lead to dizziness and a weak, washed-out feeling.

During fasting, you can't prevent the loss of sodium and water that occurs. You can and should take in some carbs (e.g., some fruit or a bit of orange juice). This limits the amount of ketosis, and can reduce the amount of salt and water loss. But the main thing you need to do is to make up for these losses by taking in about 1500–2000 mg of sodium during your OFF day. This helps keep your body salt and water content more constant and will help prevent you from feeling weak or washed out, even though you are only eating a small number of calories.

Potassium

In the last chapter, we talked about potassium and how it's very important that you keep up your potassium intake. During the OFF day, it's very difficult to take in a lot of potassium while only taking in 300–400 calories. But, if you eat mostly potassium-rich foods during the OFF day, you should still be able to take in about 2000 mg (the recommended daily amount is 4700 mg[2]). This means that most of your calories during the OFF day need to come from potassium-rich vegetables, fruits, and low-fat dairy products.

Principle 2: Drink *at least* 1000 mL (32 oz) of water

During the OFF day it's very important to drink water in addition to any other liquids that you take in. Since your kidneys will be losing both salt *and* water, to maintain the fluid spaces in your body during the OFF day, it's not enough to take in only sodium; you need to make up for the water loss as well. All food contains some water, but during the OFF day you will be eating much less food than usual, so you will need to compensate for this by drinking more water than usual. Get a large mug, fill it with bottled water, add a touch of flavor using a quarter teaspoonful (no more!) of your favorite jam and a few drops of lime juice. Sweeten it slightly, if desired, with Splenda™. Use a measuring cup so you know how many ounces or milliliters your favorite mug holds, and drink your water throughout the OFF day. Thirty-two ounces, by the way, is the minimum amount. If it is hot and you are sweating or if you exercise at all, your water needs may be higher.

Many people love to drink mineral water. Some mineral water contains up to 1800 mg/liter of bicarbonate (that's a lot!). Bicarbonate content should be listed on the label. It is not a good idea to drink high-bicarbonate mineral water when eating QOD[3]. If your favorite mineral water contains less than 250 mg/liter of bicarbonate, then it might be OK to drink a glass or two on a regular basis, but I recommend drinking mostly regular water on the OFF day.

Principle 3: Limit your food intake to 300–400 calories.

If you take in much more than 300–400 calories on your fasting day, the benefits of fasting may largely be lost. The QOD diet *may* work if you eat a few more calories than this, but the goal is to enter a fasted state during the OFF day, and also to keep your calorie intake high on the ON day so that your metabolic rate does not go down. Three to four hundred calories is a goal. You can exceed it a little bit, say to 500 calories, and still be OK, especially if you do a fair amount of walking or some exercise on the OFF day, but once you start getting up above 500 calories, you're no longer eating QOD. Try to stay at around 300–400 calories if you can.

Principle 4: Take in at least 20 g of high-biologic-value protein (from dairy, eggs or soy).

The idea here is to preserve muscle mass during weight loss Minimal daily protein requirements for people eating every day are around 50 grams per day. During the OFF day, you should eat at least 20 g of protein from dairy, eggs, or soy. Some of this you will get from your yogurt (8 oz. has 14 g). A hard-boiled egg with the yolk removed has about 4 g. So taking in some yogurt and eating 2 egg whites per day will ensure that you are taking in at least some high-biologic-value protein every day. Healthfood stores sell high-biologic-value protein powders. You can buy these and weigh out 20 g on your food scale, which is useful to do while traveling. ▓▓▓▓▓▓▓ buy a powder that is not loaded up with calories. Protein has about 4 cal/g. so 20 g of protein powder should have about 80 calories. You don't have to count these pure protein calories in the 300–400 total.

Principle 5: Take in, as supplements, fiber, calcium, and vitamins

The best situation is to get all of the fiber, calcium, and vitamins from your diet, but this is very difficult, if not impossible, to do when only eating 300–400 calories of food. So you will need to take some supplements.

Fiber supplement (8 g): One of the problems with any diet is that you may become constipated. This usually has three causes: (1) not enough fiber in the diet, (2) not enough water, and (3) not enough walking or exercise.

I recommend taking at least 8 g or more of fiber as a supplement during each OFF day. Be careful: These fiber supplements often contain substantial amounts of calories since often they are mixed with sugar or other calorie-containing substances. The fiber supplement that you choose should have no more than 20 calories per 6 g of fiber. You should not count fiber calories as part of the 300–400 daily requirement. Taking in 1000 mL of water (according to principle #2) and walking every day or doing some mild exercise will also help keep your bowel movements regular when eating QOD.

Calcium supplement (800 mg calcium): Official recommendations are that you need about 1000–1300 mg of calcium per day on average[2]. A reasonable OFF day minimum goal is 800 mg of calcium. You can't come close to this during the OFF day, however, unless you take in a calcium supplement. My favorite is calcium citrate. Usually one pill contains 200 mg of calcium, but they come in different sizes. So take enough calcium citrate supplements to give you 800 mg of calcium. Remember that you may be getting some calcium from the dairy products you will be eating as well as from calcium-fortified orange juice.

Vitamins: We talked about vitamins in the last chapter. There may be some vitamin D in your calcium supplement as well as in any dairy products you. . . . . . vitamin D is also in some, but not all, multiple vitamins. You can buy tablets of vitamin D containing 400 IU. You can take one or two of these a day, to bring your total vitamin D intake up to 800 IU per day. You may not need a vitamin D supplement if you live in an area where it is sunny and if you are out in the sun a fair amount. I recommend you take a high potency B multivitamin supplement that also contains some vitamin C during your OFF day. If you are over 50 years of age, you might consider taking, in addition, vitamin B-12. The amount you need is controversial[4] (see Appendix A).

Putting the five principles into action

What types of foods to eat

During your OFF day, you have a difficult problem—you need to take in a fairly large amount of sodium, potassium and other minerals in proportion to the amount of calories you are eating. You could take these minerals completely as supplements, but the QOD eating concept is to try to get all of the potassium and magnesium that you will need, and at least some of the calcium, from foods themselves. Why? Because these minerals are not the only ones that you need. Vegetables and fruits are naturally high in potassium and magnesium, but they also contain a host of other valuable minerals and compounds that are necessary to maintain good health; it would not be wise to deprive yourself of these other beneficial substance, even every other day. Also, taking potassium supplements without medical supervision may be dangerous.

So most of the recommended foods during the OFF day are potassium-rich, but calorie-poor, vegetables and fruits. There also is room for low-fat dairy products, as discussed below.

1. Liquid foods: Tomato-vegetable juice, orange juice, and liquid yogurt:

My own recommended approach is to rely to a great extent on eating three liquid foods during the OFF day: tomato-vegetable juice (e.g., V-8™, a product that contains tomato juice plus seven other vegetable juices[5]), orange juice, and liquid yogurt. Why? One advantage is that they are widely available. If you need to be on the QOD diet while traveling, or are rushing off to work and missed breakfast, these products can be found at most local grocery stores or gas stations.

These three foods are different in terms of the sodium, potassium, calcium and calories they contain, and you need to understand how they differ to use them most effectively.

a) Tomato-vegetable juice: 6 calories/oz; lots of sodium and potassium

Tomato juice is a great food for the OFF day. Why? Because it has very few calories, but is loaded with potassium, and also has lots of sodium (you can buy low-sodium tomato juice, but I don't recommend this for the OFF day). You can buy tomato (or tomato-vegetable) juice either in bottles or cans. I don't recommend buying aluminum cans, because in the past there have been reports of aluminum leaching from aluminum cookware into foods containing tomato sauces. The aluminum cans may be safe, but why take the risk?

Tomato-vegetable juice: Serving size: 8 oz (240 ml)
Calories: 50   Sodium: 600 mg   Potassium: 480 mg   Carbs: 8 g

---

The nice thing about tomato-vegetable juice is, after drinking 8 oz (240 mL), you've taken care of about ⅓ of your daily sodium goal and almost ¼ of your daily potassium goal, and you've only ingested 50 calories.

One company now makes several versions of tomato-vegetable juice (V-8™) to vary the taste a bit. One version comes with added zesty spices ("spicy hot"), and another with lemon juice. A calcium- and potassium-supplemented variety (V-8™ Bone Health™) also is available. Diluting tomato or veggie juice with water may improve its taste for people who find it too concentrated or salty. If you like tomato juice or V-8™, it will be much easier for you to stay on the QOD diet.

b) Orange juice: 14 calories/oz; lots of potassium, (when. . . .ted) lots of calcium, no sodium.

Orange juice is a great food because it has a lot of potassium, but at 14 calories/oz, it has more than twice the calories of tomato juice.

Orange Juice: Serving size: 8 oz (240 ml)
Calories: 110   Sodium: 0 mg   Potassium: 450 mg   Carbs: 26 g

---

An 8-oz serving of orange juice has 26 g of carbs, three times that of tomato juice, so I recommend taking it in small amounts (4 oz half-serving, containing 55 calories) first thing in the morning and whenever you feel you need some carbs. Some types of orange juice are now supplemented with calcium and vitamin D and you can get up to 35% of your daily requirement of calcium from an 8-oz glass. Orange juice has no sodium, so you will have to get sodium elsewhere.

c) Drinkable yogurt: 10–14 calories/oz; lots of potassium, lots of calcium, low in sodium.

A third liquid food that I use a lot when eating QOD is drinkable yogurt. Don't confuse this with regular, flavored yogurts that usually are loaded with sugar. One Chicago-area company, Lifeway Foods, makes two varieties of unflavored, drinkable yogurt. They call them Kefir and Kwashenka. The two are quite similar, but they have a slightly different taste. Low-fat Kwashenka is the one I like in particular. Plain only, please. Stay away from the flavored varieties.

Drinkable Yogurt (plain): Serving size: 8 oz (240 ml)

Calories:	Sodium:	Potassium:	Carbs:
110 (low-fat)	125 mg	480 mg	8 g
85 (non-fat)			
Calcium 30%			

There are several nice things about drinkable yogurt. First of all, tomato and orange juice have almost no protein or fat. Drinkable yogurt has at least some protein and, if you get the low fat version, at least a bit of fat. More importantly, drinkable yogurt can be enjoyed by itself, flavored with some Splenda™ and cinnamon. In addition, drinkable yogurt can be made into a dressing to be poured over fruit, or made into a low calorie sauce to be used as a raw vegetable dip, steamed vegetable sauce, or salad dressing.

So the way to stay healthy and feel good during the OFF day is to take in a substantial amount of each of these three basic liquid foods. Now, if you are counting calories, you can see that if you drink two 8-oz servings of tomato-vegetable juice, that's already 100 calories. If you then add 4 oz of orange juice and 4 oz of drinkable yogurt, that's another 50 or so calories each, and you're already up to about 200 calories. So you only have 100 calories left (200 if you're going up to 400 calories a day) for other foods. This doesn't leave a lot of room for snacking on the side or cheating during the OFF day.

Measuring cup: Those of you who cook will know what this is and how to use it—those of you who don't may have never seen one. Measuring cups are marked off in terms of cups, ounces, or milliliters (mL). When you drink tomato juice, orange juice or liquid yogurt during your OFF day, be sure to measure out the amounts, so that you don't exceed the goal amount of calories. Mark your favorite mugs so that you know how much 4, 8, and 12 oz are.

2. Solid food mini-meals

Most of the solid foods you will be eating during the OFF day should be vegetables and small helpings of certain fruits.

Vegetable mini-meals:

There are three ways you can prepare and eat vegetables: as a crunchy finger food, in salads, and served hot (steamed, pan-fried or microwaved).

Crunchy finger food: The French have a term for this: *amuse-bouche.* Foods that amuse your mouth! You always need a plate of these in the refrigerator or on the countertop through-out the . . . . naine lettuce leaves are great for this, as are celery sticks and radishes. Also, try slices of green or red pepper or zucchini. Cucumbers may be the best, as well as small, cherry tomatoes. You can use drinkable yogurt to make a dipping sauce (with lime juice and salt), but again, measure everything out and count the calories. Here's another idea: You can buy low-calorie salsa dip, 10 calories per tablespoon (15 mL). Take two table-spoons and pour into 2 or 3 Romaine lettuce leaves. Fold over and eat your "lettuce tacos". To help guide you, in Appendix B, we have photos of 25-calorie portions of some common crunchy vegetables.

Salads: Here you have a lot of choices. Salads have few calo-ries. You can make one using lettuce or spinach, tomatoes, pick-les (especially if you need a little salt), cucumbers, green peppers, radishes, and whatever else crosses your mind. Ideally, you should weigh your salad after making it using a food scale (see below). Most salad-type vegetables have about 0.2 calories per gram. So a 25-calorie salad should weigh no more than about 130 grams. Please be careful about store-bought salad dressing, as this usually has about 40 calories per tablespoon. It is much better to make a salad dressing from drinkable yogurt (4–7 calories per tablespoon, instead!). You can add some salt, dill, lemon juice, and other spices to taste. Then you can use 2 oz of this dressing (60 mL, or 4 tablespoons), and you will have used up only 25 calories or so. Please, no croutons, bacon bits or almonds. Otherwise your salad can climb to several hundred calories.

One of my favorite salads is made by cutting up one or two small tomatoes, two small pickles, some onions, and garnishing with a yogurt dressing. If I have a few calories left to eat, I add a few small pieces of cheese.

Hot vegetable dishes: These are easy to prepare from either raw vegetables or from frozen food packs. Some vegetables can have a fair number of calories, though, and should be eaten very sparingly. Potatoes are out. Corn and lima beans have a lot of calories. Carrots and peas are intermediate. Among the best choices are green beans, squash, and zucchini. Before preparing, check the nutrition labels and make sure that the amount you are preparing does not exceed 25–50 calories. When heating your vegetables, frying in oil is out, although you can use spray-on oil. You can steam asparagus or zucchini in a skillet using a small amount of water, and you can also use a tiny amount of oil to pan fry some garlic or onions for taste. Steamed asparagus with oregano and spices garnished with yogurt sauce is one of my favorite dishes.

Fruit mini-meals:

Here you have to be quite careful, since many fruits have a lot of calories. At least the first time, you need to check calorie counts and either weigh out the fruits or count out the berries so that you don't go over your calorie limit. Blueberries, raspberries, or strawberries, or a few slices of apple, plum or peach, topped with drinkable yogurt and sweetened with Splenda™ makes a delicious treat. Appendix B shows 25-calorie portions of some common fruits: you can combine any of these with 2 oz of drinkable yogurt (60mL, 25 calories) to make a 50-calorie mini-meal, or you can just snack on the fruits by themselves without any topping. Sprinkling slices of apple or peach with cinnamon and Splenda™ can give them a nice taste.

3. **Solid foods to eat in very small quantities (meats, nuts, fats, oils, butter)**

Here you're sort of stuck. These foods are healthy for you as part of a balanced diet, but you need to save them for the ON days. Even small amounts of these foods can add up to quite a few calories, and this will cause you to go well over your 300–400 calorie daily limit. For example, if you look in Appendix B, you will find that most vegetables that we are recommending contain 0.2 to 0.5 calories per gram. Fruits are about 0.6 calories per gram. On the other hand, most meats are about 4 calories per gram, and nuts are 5 calories per gram. This means that 2 or 3 shelled walnuts will make a 25 calorie mini-meal, or about five peanuts. Sometimes, though you get a strong craving for something other than fruits or vegetables. Then a few peanuts (about 5 calories per shelled peanut), a quarter teaspoon of peanut butter, or a small ultra-thin piece of salami may make your OFF day easier. If you sense that you need some protein, hard boil two eggs and remove the yolks. Eat the whites only (flavored with a bit of spaghetti sauce or ketchup). Each egg white contains only 17–20 calories and has 4–5 g of protein. Protein is also found in diary products: Half a piece of processed cheese has about 25–40 calories. This has more calories and fat than yogurt, but sometimes you will just feel the need for a bit of cheese.

In general you should avoid eating bread on your OFF day. Bread just has too many calories. You can have a few chips or crackers. Usually crackers are 10–20 calories each, depending on size. Most potato chips are about 10 calories a chip. Bread group foods have important nutrients, but the amount of potassium they contain per calorie is much lower than vegetables and fruits. You will need to put off eating meat, oils and breads until the ON day (fortunately, it's just one day away!).

Learning how to count calories and use a digital food scale

To eat during the OFF day and lose weight, you will need to stay within the calorie goals. To do this, you will have to take some time and learn about how many calories (as well as potassium) typical foods contain. A number of websites can show you this. The websites that I recommend can be reached via *eatQOD.com*. There you will be able to find how many calories are in whatever type of food you may desire.

One problem with calories on food labels, and even from websites, is that the number of calories is listed in terms of portion size, or, on the website, in terms of sizes of food. What is a slice of bread? How big is a medium apple or a glass of orange juice? If you're eating 2000 calories per day, a small mistake in terms of portion size is trivial, but when you're serious about eating only 300–400 calories a day, you need to know fairly exactly how many calories are in the food that you're eating. The best way to do this is to get a good scale. The one that I use and recommend is manufactured by a company called Soehnle. They make several types of scales, ranging in price from about $20 to $80. The digital food scale I use is the Soehnle Myra Digital Food Scale, which costs about $29.99 plus shipping from *amazon.com*.

Once you have a food scale, you should begin to educate yourself about how many calories are contained in the fruits and vegetables that you will be eating. For example, you may like apples. How many calories in an apple? From a calorie-counting website, you might learn that a "large" apple has 110 calories, but what does this mean? Looking further, you find that such an apple should weigh 212 grams. But how much does *your* apple weigh? You take it out of the refrigerator and weigh it, and you may find that *your* apple weighs 270 grams, and so has about 30% more calories than listed.

What to drink (other than water)

Principle #2 for the OFF day is to take in 32 oz of water. This is in addition to the tomato and orange juice and liquid yogurt that you take in. Additional drinks you might try are tea, coffee, or hot chocolate (made with unsweetened cocoa and sweetened with Splenda™.) I recommend avoiding all presweetened diet sodas.

If you drink coffee on a regular basis, you should continue to drink it (maximum of 2 cups) during your OFF day. Coffee should not count as part of your water intake. In fact, coffee acts on the kidneys to increase salt and water loss in the urine, which you are trying to minimize during the OFF day. So this is a minus. On the plus side, caffeine has a tendency to increase the metabolic rate, which can be useful while dieting. Also, withdrawal headaches can sometimes occur in people who suddenly stop their habitual coffee intake. Be careful about adding lots of milk or creamer to your coffee—that can quickly drive up the total number of calories.

A brief walk through a typical OFF day.

When you ⸺ ⸺ the morning of an OFF day, you really shouldn't be hungry. Many people are typically not very hungry at breakfast time anyway. One reason is that even during the "fast" of sleeping overnight, they are beginning to move slightly into ketosis.

Now, if you try to eat nothing at all when you wake up, by lunchtime you may not be feeling very well. For one thing, you'll have already lost some salt. So don't skip eating in the morning—you need some food, some salt, and a considerable amount of water. The ideal "breakfast" is a glass (8 oz) of tomato juice or veggie juice (50 calories), a cup of coffee (0 calories) and maybe some snack vegetables or fruit (25 calories). It's very important to remember to drink 32 oz of water throughout the day, and your first 12 oz should be ingested as soon as you get up in morning. The morning food intake should include at least 500 mg of sodium. In the morning, it's also wise to take half of your calcium citrate supplements (Personally, I split the calcium supplement intake between a morning and an afternoon dose.) plus maybe an additional 400 IU of vitamin D, plus your B-complex multivitamins with C, and also 8 g or more of fiber supplement.

If you get to lunchtime and start feeling slightly weak, don't hesitate to take a second glass of tomato juice *and* at least 12 oz of water. Many people are surprised by how satisfying one simple glass of (high-sodium) veggie juice plus water can be. It can be as satiating as a good spaghetti dinner. If you still feel you need salt, eat a sliced up pickle and drink 12 oz of water.

By suppertime, if you haven't had a chance to take in your recommended sodium, potassium, or water intake, you should correct that now. Around 5–7 PM, you should prepare and eat your main solid meal of the day, and it should consist mostly of prepared vegetables and fruits, as described above. A hot vegetable dish may be the most satisfying.

If you find hunger in the evening a problem, again you assuage it depending on what the problem is. Salt or potassium craving? More tomato juice (or tomato paste spread on some vegetables can work). Need for something to munch on? Try some snack vegetables, especially lettuce leaves, celery, or radishes. Feel like you need some carbs? Half a glass (measured, 4 oz, or 120 mL) of orange juice. Need fat? Four or five peanuts or a ¼ teaspoon of peanut butter will often do the trick and make you feel better. Need protein? Try some egg whites or some yogurt.

During the OFF day, you should be taking in sufficient carbs to prevent a high degree of ketosis, but some people will still get a mild ketosis. If this causes discomfort, taking in some orange juice helps the body continue to burn some carbs.

Generally, you shouldn't eat anything much after about 8 PM during the OFF day, but remember to keep up your water intake. It's recommended to take in a 12 oz glass of water before going to bed. This helps keep up your body water stores during the night and also helps keep the kidneys working. You can heat this water up and add a ¼ teaspoonful of your favorite jam and some Splenda™ to make a home-made, caffeine-free tea.

OFF-Day Eating for Real People in Real-World Situations

The OFF day does have its rewards, but it also holds challenges. One of the more difficult among these is the issue of dealing with social eating situations.

Just because you're on the QOD diet doesn't mean the rest of the world is going to join you! Your coworkers and business colleagues—even your family—will go right on eating every day as they always have.

So what do you do when you have a business lunch that you really have to attend? Or a company party? What about the family dinner? Celebrating a birthday?

Well, first of all, your decision to follow the QOD diet doesn't mean you're the first and only employee in human history who has ever gone on a diet. People do it all the time—including people who have jobs. And it's the most normal thing in the world for people who are dieting to explain what they're doing to their coworkers, and to firmly but politely decline when it's time to eat.

If you're at a business lunch, you can order some water to drink plus tomato juice. Diet soda in this case is OK, but you will need to get your sodium and potassium from somewhere. You can order a small salad, but always ask that the salad dressing be brought on the side instead of mixed with the salad, so that you can add it yourself. Remember that the usual salad dressings typically have 40 or more calories per tablespoon! Stay away from the bread rolls and butter. For social reasons, you may need to eat something in addition. If this becomes necessary, then eat as small an amount as you can from what you have ordered.

At a party or celebration, the goodies are usually spread out on tables, and you may find a veggie tray you can pick from or maybe even a tossed salad if it hasn't been pre-loaded with dressing and croutons.

What about at home? If you are in the habit of sitting down at mealtimes with your family, of course you don't want to change that. Have a glass of water and one of your glasses of tomato juice, and some raw veggies that you've prepared ahead of time to store in the fridge. You can steam up your own vegetable mini-meal, or eat a small amount of the vegetables being served. Enjoy the conversation. If there's something that's passed around the table that looks particularly tempting (like rack of ribs!) just put your portion aside in the fridge so you can enjoy it the next day. If it's a birthday, and you just can't refuse a piece of little Tommy's birthday cake, then go ahead and cut a small piece. Eat it slowly. After all, how often do birthdays happen?

Rewards Await on Your OFF day

With a little planning and some definite commitment, those OFF days when you fast shouldn't pose a major problem for you.

Now, if before this, you've associated the words *fast* and *fasting* with deprivation, discomfort, and intense hunger, it's time to change your thinking. For one thing, if you follow the principles and guidelines in this book, your OFF days really won't be unbearable and so unpleasant you have to call on your last ounce of willpower just to make it through the day. You won't grow weak and listless, and you certainly aren't going to waste away and become gaunt and emaciated.

So banish those images and thoughts from ~~your mind~~. Think of your OFF days instead as opportunities to retrain your appetite, to give your digestive system a much-needed rest, and to get in touch with what your body really wants and needs to best nourish itself. Remind yourself that you are learning to eat with conscious awareness instead of mindlessly reaching for food out of habit or to assuage a carb craving.

There's another reward that's yours for taking every other day "off" from eating regular meals, and that's a savings of time. Eating does take time, and there's also food preparation time—even if it's making peanut butter and jelly sandwiches and packing a lunch. Preparing a full evening meal can take far more time. Then there's the cleanup: Clearing the table, storing the leftovers, loading the dishwasher—all this too takes time. Even driving to a restaurant and back takes time. During your OFF day, you save all of this time normally spent in food preparation, eating, and cleanup. This time saved

---

OFF day eating guide summary:

Goals:

300–400 calories

1500–2000[1] mg sodium, 2000 mg potassium, 32 oz (1000 mL) water

8 g fiber supplements, 800 mg calcium supplements plus vitamins

20 g of high-biologic-value protein

---

can be a benefit to you if you put it to good use. What will you do with it all?

You want to think about this carefully. Because if all this extra time just winds up hanging in front of you like an empty sack with nothing to fill it, then you'll be far more likely to spend some of it "monitoring" how you feel. Was that a hunger pang? Am I in discomfort? What if I can't make it through the day? Maybe I should head over and r.　　　 :. the refrigerator.

When you fill up the time you're saving with activities that you enjoy and that capture your attention, your mind will be diverted from fretting about your physical sensations. You'll be far more likely to succeed in eating QOD if you plan ahead to spend this time gained on some worthwhile pursuits. You could take a walk, pick up a neglected hobby, do some journaling, or head for the gym to work out. You could register for an evening class, do some community volunteer work, do some repairs around the house, or clean the garage or attic. With a little creative thought, you'll come up with plenty of things you've wished you *could* do—or known you *should* do—but for which you never before could seem to find the time.

Remember, Relief is a Day Away

One great advantage of the QOD diet is that when you come to an OFF day, it's not as if you're now swearing off food for the rest of your life. You don't have to resign yourself to deprivation and sacrifice and discomfort for the duration of your diet. No, satisfaction is never more than a day away. Focus your mind not on what you're giving up, but on what you're getting in return. Not on self-pity but on self-congratulation.

Here's a hot tip (veggie juice soup):

Boil up your favorite veggie juice in a pot. Add some diced garlic, onions, and/or celery and maybe a small piece of cheese. Simmer. Flavor with basil, pepper, and Splenda.™

One measure of maturity is the ability to delay gratification—to sacrifice a little here and now for a future reward. The QOD diet will help you build more self-discipline—without stretching you far beyond your comfort zone. Most of us don't get many chances to build this kind of discipline, so look on this as contributing to your self-development.

Calories	Meals
	Breakfast:
50	Tomato juice: 8 oz
50	Orange juice: 4 oz
	Lunch:
50	Tomato juice: 8 oz
25	One fruit or vegetable snack or salad
25	Drinkable yogurt (2 oz) as a dressing for above
	Mini-snack (anytime):
25	Crunchy vegetable mini-meal
	Dinner:
25–50	Hot vegetable plate (zucchini, green beans, asparagus, squash)
25	Yogurt dressing
50	Egg whites (2) plus tomato dressing
	Evening:
25	Orange juice (4 oz) if you feel need for more carbs.
375	**Total**

Snack calories (25–50, or a bit more if you are exercising):

Any fruit: 0.6 cal/g	10 calories = 16 g
Vegetables: 0.2–0.8 cal/g	10 calories = about 25 g
Most meats and breads and chips:	4 cal/gram 10 calories = 2.5 g
Fatty foods (walnuts): 5+ cal/g	10 calories = about 2 g

CHAPTER 6

THE ON DAY: HOW YOU SHOULD EAT
(AND HOW YOU SHOULDN'T)

S o you've finished with your OFF day yesterday and now it's morning, and—it's an ON day! How much should you eat? When should you eat, and what foods should you eat?

This chapter too will present principles (five of them, again) to assist you in making eating during your ON days as effective and pleasant as possible.

Principle 1: How much should you eat? *Eat within reason, 5–6 medium-sized meals, without gluttony or binging.*

Eating well is different from eating like crazy. The QOD diet helps the metabolic rate stay up, but to lose weight, you still need to eat fewer calories on average than what your body requires to maintain its weight. Because this amount of calories is fairly high, I don't recommend using food scales or calorie counters.

That being said, it's useful to know about how many calories you should be eating to achieve weight loss. The calculations, for those who are interested, are discussed in more detail in Appendix

A[1]. After you go through all of the equations and tables, you almost always will come up with a goal ON day calorie intake between 2000 and 2600 calories. The main differences are due to gender, height and activity level. Assuming a normal level of activity, for a shorter woman, the ON day calorie goal would be 2000 calories per day. For a taller man, the ON day goal is around 2600 calories. So that's about how much you should be eating.

No binging or gluttony; eat small, frequen ile you should be able to eat pretty much what you want on your ON day, you should avoid making it a "pig-out" day. After fasting for one full day, you might think that you would end up so terribly hungry the next day that you would be unable to keep yourself from vacuuming up all the food your eyes can see. At least one research study suggests that this doesn't happen: After a 36-hour fast, people did not compensate by overeating.[2]

The potentially serious dangers of eating large meals have been described in Chapter 2 and Appendix A. Large meals may be associated with an increased risk of heart attack, and also can cause low blood pressure. So avoid taking in very large meals and eat many small or medium-sized meals throughout the day. Eat well but *within reason*, and put on the brakes before you reach gluttony.

After your medium-sized meal, stop eating for 1–2 hours, even if you're still hungry: Remember, you're listening to your body now for specific hungers, but it takes some time for the food you eat to "register". So you listen, and your body is telling you, "Wally, I'm hungry for walnuts", or "Bart, I need some bananas". So you start eating walnuts or bananas. Half-an-hour later, your body is saying, "Still hungry for walnuts or bananas". The problem is, that the walnuts or bananas are still in your stomach and haven't been absorbed yet. Especially if you eat quickly, you might eat more walnuts or bananas than you really want or need. So after you've eaten a medium-sized meal, even if you're still hungry, wait a bit and let this food be absorbed before you decide you want to eat again.

Principle 2: When to eat: *Breakfast is the most important meal: Make sure to eat a substantial breakfast (including water and 500 mg of sodium) soon after you get up.*

The morning of your ON day, you would think that you would be starved and hungry enough to eat a huge breakfast. For some reason (it may have to do with ketosis), many people aren't that hungry when they get up on the ON day. The first thing you should do on arising is to drink a ... (... oz) glass of water, and take in some food containing at least 500 mg of sodium. *Even if you're not hungry,* you should make sure to eat a medium-sized breakfast within half an hour or so of getting up. Remember, you are breaking the fast with this meal. The goal is to make sure that your body sodium and water contents stay up—or, if these have dropped slightly after 36 hours of partial fasting, to get them back up to normal as soon as possible. Usually, eating a breakfast that contains 500 mg of sodium is no problem. One bagel has 540 mg of sodium. A slice of bread with some mayonnaise and cheese will meet the requirement easily. If for some reason you need to rush out to work or to an appointment, drink 12-oz of tomato-vegetable juice and a large glass of water as you are running out the door.

There may be some general health and weight-loss advantages to shifting your daily calorie intake around so that you eat a substantial amount of your food in the morning. For example, research shows that if you're among those who typically skip breakfast, and then you begin to include a good breakfast, that one change alone can help you lose weight. Research also suggests that eating breakfast helps reduce dietary fat consumption and also impulsive snacking.[3]

Principle 3: When to eat: *Space out 5–6 medium-sized meals throughout the day.*

Proper spacing of meals during the ON day is very important. You should eat at least 5–6 times during the ON day. One to two hours after eating breakfast, you may get quite hungry again. This is fine—eat a mid-morning snack. You should take in about ¼ of your calories between 7 AM (assuming that's when you arise) and 11 AM.

How to space out your food intake	
Time	**% calories**
7 AM–11 AM	25%
11 AM–4 PM (two meals!)	50%
4 PM–8 PM (two meals)	25%

Then you should be eating ½ of your daily intake (at least two divided meals) between 11 AM and 4 PM. You will be hungry, but listen carefully to your body and eat those foods that you are hungry for. Finally, the remaining ¼ of your food intake should come in the early evening, from 4 PM to 8 PM, again, in 2 medium-sized meals.

Do all you can to avoid eating a big, late supper. Many Americans have fallen into the habit of eating only a very small breakfast—or even no breakfast at all—then a small lunch, and finally a very large evening meal. They come home from work, eat a big, late meal around 8 or 9 PM, then feel so tired they just "veg" out in front of the TV for a while before heading for bed. When they lie down for the night, that large meal gets the stomach acids churning, and while sleeping, the acid backs up into the esophagus. This creates esophagitis, heartburn and can eventually can result in acid reflux disease. The dangers of large meals have been discussed above. So it's important to keep all of the meals during your ON day moderate in size.

Principle 4: What to eat: Choose a healthy balance of foods and avoid very high sodium foods

What sorts of foods should you eat during your ON day? All cake and donuts? Obviously not. Low-fat diet? No. Low-carb diet? No. What should be the ideal proportion of carbs, fats, and protein? The latest guidelines were discussed in Chapter 4 (you can read these at *health.gov/dietaryguidelines/*
and at *iom.edu/Object.File/Master/21/372/0.pdf*)[1].
These suggest that adults should be eating about 20–35% of their calories as fats, 45–65% as carbs, and 10–35% as protein. There is no reason to depart from this sound advice.

Apart from breakfast, there is no reason to keep a high sodium intake during your ON day. In fact, you want your kidneys to get used to a smaller sodium load. So try and avoid processed and salty foods during lunch and supper. You want to stay close to recommended amounts of total sodium intake (see Chapter 2) during the ON day.

You want to eat lots and lots of vegetables and fruits to make sure you get enough potassium during your ON day, but you also need your proteins and fats and bread group foods. Remember, during your OFF day, almost all of your calories came from carbs. So the ON day is also the time to enjoy the benefits of eating meat, fish, nuts and unsaturated fats, as well as breads and pasta made with whole grains.

What about desserts? Why not? A donut? Go for it. But limit yourself to one dessert (normal portion size, now—don't cheat!) during the ON day.

Principle 5: What to eat: Listen to your body's specific food hungers

One of the chief goals of undertaking the QOD diet is to train yourself to listen to your body to figure out what it needs. As we've noted before, so many Americans just eat mindlessly, letting taste or advertising or "what looks good" dictate their food choices. And without making deliberate, conscious choices, it's all too easy to follow the path of least resistance and end up habitually choosing foods high in fat as well as sugar and other highly refined carbs.

Eating QOD helps break the cycle of mindless eating. For perhaps the first time ever, you'll learn that, when given a chance, your body will actually "speak" to you in the form of hunger—not for just "food" in general, but for specific foods. It may take a while to begin hearing what your body has to say, but rest assured that as you continue to build in those every-other-day breaks from eating, your body will begin suggesting to you what it craves.

When that happens, listen carefully. On your ON days, if you are not really hungry for a particular food, don't eat it. If you are, then go for it. You may want to eat just a serving of corn or peas or a leg of chicken and nothing else. Hungry for fat? Try walnuts or some food containing vegetable oil such as mayonnaise. Carbs? Bananas are great, as is orange juice. Protein? How about some eggs or some meat or fish?

In the event that your body doesn't seem to be telegraphing its hunger for anything specific, then at least make a healthful choice. Choose a handful of nuts as a snack and don't jump first to a high-carb, high-fat choice (like a cookie or pastry). Always have some fresh veggie snacks, salads, nuts, and fruits in the fridge. Again, stocking your kitchen properly is so important: If you get hungry for, peas or corn, but the only food you have in house is chips and hot-dogs, then chips and dogs is what you'll wind up eating, and what's worse, your specific hunger will remain unassuaged.

> Tip: You're traveling or have no good access to food and it's an ON day. Buy some veggie juice to start off the day, and then buy some trail mix and bottled water. Snack on the trail mix (a mixture of peanuts, other nuts, and fruits) to get in at least 1000 calories of food during that part of the day when you don't have time to eat a regular meal and make sure you also drink at least 32 oz of water.

Additional suggestions:

Water: Finally, don't forget to keep up with your water intake. You will be taking in more water as part of your food on the ON day, but it is still easy to get a bit dehydrated. In particular, you don't want to overeat because you think you're hungry, when you really were mostly thirsty.

Fiber and other supplements: I still recommend taking at least 8 g of fiber supplement during the ON day, as well as some calcium, some vitamin D, and also, B and C vitamins. You will be eating a normal diet so B and C vitamin supplements may not be necessary, but I still recommend them, according to the information supplied in Chapter 2.

Summing up:

If you follow these five principles, you'll come to genuinely enjoy those ON days. Your food will taste better. You'll learn to tune in to your body's messages. You'll break free of enslavement by unhealthy food cravings. And—best of all, you'll see the results on your scale and in the ever-loosening fit of your clothes.

CHAPTER 7

MONITORING, PROBLEMS, AND THEIR SOLUTIONS

OK, now that you've begun QOD, how do you stay on track? What should you monitor, and how often? At what speed should you be losing weight? What are the common problems and how can you solve them? How can you modify the basic QOD plan if you need to?

Weighing yourself twice a day

Some diet plans recommend that you weigh yourself every day; others that you don't focus on weighing yourself and only check your weight once a week or so. Normally your weight will fluctuate quite a bit during each day and also from day to day. I recommend that you weigh yourself twice a day, once on just getting up, and once before going to bed using a digital scale. You will find that your weight will vary within a given day by as much as 4 pounds, and will always be lowest in the morning. When eating QOD, your weight will be lowest on the morning of your ON day. Since your weight will jump around so much, it will be difficult to know whether you are making progress unless you graph your weight and take a 4-day moving average. I have provided a tool that you can use on my website: *eatQOD.com*. You can log in and chart your weights there using a calendar tool, and then you can print out and save a graph of your progress. Here is what one such graph looks like:

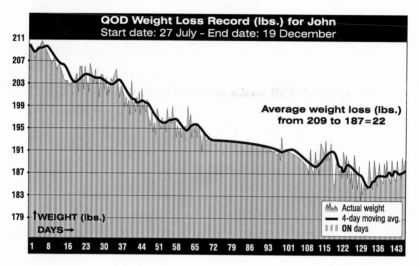

In this case, QOD eating was started on July 27 (day 1). About 22 lbs were lost over the next 120 days (4 months). You can see that the weight loss tended to be greatest during the first 2 weeks, (days 1–16) then stabilized for about 2 more weeks, and then resumed. This happens with diets. Sometimes, even when looking at a 4-day average curve, weight loss will stop for a week or two, and then start up again.

Why is body weight always lower in the morning? There are four reasons: (1) The main one has to do with metabolism of your glycogen stores, which contain a lot of water. (2) You continue to lose water (not only from glycogen metabolism but also from other sources) in your breath during the night. (3) Your kidneys tend to excrete more salt and water as you change from metabolism of glucose to burning ketones. (4) When you lay down, your legs are up relatively high in relation to your heart, and this increases blood return to the heart and indirectly, to the kidneys.

How much weight should you be losing? Most diet experts agree that losing a pound a week, or 4 lbs. per month, is a good pace for weight loss. In the graph above, over 122 days, 22 lbs were lost, so the average weight loss was about 5 lbs per month.

QOD problems and their solutions

Weakness and lightheadedness. When this happens it's usually on the evening of the OFF day or the morning of the ON day. The cause can be either sodium and water loss or a need for carbs. **Drink more water:** First of all, make sure that you are drinking at least 32 oz of water on your OFF day. **Caffeinated beverages:** Avoid caffeinated drinks in the afternoon or evening of your OFF day. Caffeine acts like a water pill and tends to dry you out. **Sodium and carbs:** If weakness is a problem, the best thing to do is to drink some tomato-vegetable juice and/or orange juice when this happens. If this is happening mostly during the ON day morning, take 4 oz of tomato juice and 4 oz of orange juice in the evening of the OFF day. The tomato juice will help keep more salt and water in your system, and orange juice will lower the amount of ketosis during the night.

As a last ditch effort, you might try to increase your calorie intake a bit during the OFF day to 500 calories a day. These "cheater calories" should be mostly orange juice or other carbs, and they should be taken toward the evening of the OFF day. In this event you should try some low intensity exercise like walking or slow swimming to help you burn the extra OFF day calories.

It's important to know that the QOD diet is NOT for everyone. If you do follow this advice and still don't feel strong or well, then QOD eating is not for you.

Severe, gnawing hunger pangs and *Helicobacter*

You shouldn't get severe hunger pangs during the OFF day. There may be a feeling of some gurgling in the stomach area and some very mild hunger pangs—this is normal and is due to the stomach contracting a bit, since it isn't constantly being distended with food. If you develop a fairly intense pain or gnawing discomfort in the abdomen (sometimes this pain is felt in the upper back) each time you stop eating for even a few hours, and if this pain tends to be relieved when you eat, you may have peptic ulcer disease. This is due to the stomach making too much gastric acid. Another clue is, if you smoke the gnawing hunger pains get worse. People who have too much acid secretion in their stomach may be may be infected with a bacterium called *Helicobacter pylori*. This little bug infects the lining of the stomach and irritates it, making the stomach pump out acid even when acid is not needed for digestion.

If you try QOD and start getting marked pain or gnawing in the upper abdomen (or sometimes the back) after not eating for a few hours, you should stop the QOD diet and seek medical help. Fortunately, it's very easy to get rid of *Helicobacter pylori* infection if you have this. The treatment is fairly simple—two or three antibiotics plus a pill that cuts down gastric acid secretion, taken for 7–14 days. Sometimes Pepto-Bismol™ is added. Once *Helicobacter pylori* has been eradicated, it usually does not come back, and many people have less gastric upset and distress after treatment. If such is the case, you might try the QOD diet again once your *Helicobacter pylori* infection has been eradicated.

Burning pains in the upper stomach and lower chest (acid reflux): The first step is to see your doctor. Pain in this area can be due to many things—including cardiac pain. The pain may be due to acid reflux. Acid reflux usually is due to stomach acid percolating up and irritating the esophagus. One common cause is eating too much food too late in the day. When you lay down to sleep at night, all of this food stimulates your stomach to secrete acid-containing digestive juices, which then can irritate your esophagus. If this pain is due to acid reflux, try to eat very little after about 7 PM on the ON day. You may need to take in some carbs or sodium-containing foods to feel better, but avoid having a full meal.

Eating too much during the ON day: One problem associated with any diet is, that diets can train people to focus too much on food, and because people can get very hungry, any diet can increase the tendency for people to binge eat. You should gain 2–4 lbs during a typical ON day. If you find yourself regularly gaining more, this may be a sign of binge eating, and you should stop the QOD diet right away.

Getting to like fasting too much: Eating QOD is a way to fast and not feel too badly, since mineral balance is maintained. You may be tempted to fast for more than one day in a row. This is a bad idea. First of all, your body will quickly lower its metabolic rate, and you will need to stay at a very low calorie intake to lose weight. Secondly, the intake of nutrients and minerals during an OFF day, while better than nothing, is far from optimal. You can get away with it if you're eating QOD, because you are eating well during your ON day. So it's not a good idea to fast for more than one day at a time. Also, if you find that you're developing a tendency toward anorexia, stop eating QOD right away.

Constipation: This will tend to happen if you don't take at least 8 g of a fiber supplement during your OFF day. You may need more to stay regular. Also, remember the importance of an adequate water intake and walking or other exercise. Calcium supplements can be constipating, but you need your calcium. So take your fiber supplements, drink your water, and walk every day or exercise, and constipation shouldn't be a problem.

If you don't like tomato juice: Some people who hate tomato juice have tried to go on the QOD diet, and it's been difficult for them. There are no alternative vegetable juices readily available that have the nutrient profile of tomato juice or tomato-vegetable juice. The company that makes V-8 does make it in several "flavors", and this helps with variety. If you can't stand tomato juice, you will need to get your potassium and other minerals normally found here somewhere else and you will have to be careful not to overdose on sodium. Alternate sources of sodium include pickles, soy sauce, and just plain salt. be careful when using salt from the shaker (a ¼ teaspoon contains about 560 mg of sodium), because if you're off by a bit you can wind up eating way too much sodium. Buy and use little salt packets (the kind they use in restaurants) so that you know exactly how much salt you're taking in. It is very important to take in at least 2000 mg of potassium during the OFF day. *It is not health-*

ful nor wise to take in sodium during the OFF day, but to avoid tak-ing in the recommended amounts of potassium and magnesium.

The easiest substitute for tomato juice is tomato paste or toma-toes. You can weigh out 250 g of tomatoes, and this has the same amount of calories, potassium and other minerals as 8-oz of tomato juice. Tomato paste comes both salted and unsalted. You can spread this on your crunchy vegetables, and calculate the potassium content from the calories counter websites available via *eatQC* ˙ner thing to try: Try boiling up the tomato-based veggie juice as a soup and add vegetables (celery, onions) and flavor (pepper, Splenda™) to taste.

How to do this with no tomatoes at all? Two 8-oz servings of tomato juice contain 1000–1300 mg of potassium, so you need to get this some other way. You can drink more orange juice, or other potassium-rich fruit juices such as kiwi or papaya juice, but you will also be increasing your calories and even more so, your OFF day carbs. Also, these other juices are not so widely available. It might be easiest to eat a lot of potassium-rich vegetables, but then you have to plan ahead and keep a stock of these available. Lists of such vegeta-bles are available at *eatQOD.com*.

Lower-sodium versions of QOD eating

The main reason for taking in 1500–2000 mg of sodium during the OFF day is to keep sodium intake about the same as it is during your ON day. Some people like to follow a much lower sodium diet. If you are one of these, then you can try switching to low-sodium tomato or tomato-vegetable juice during the OFF day. Myself, I love the taste of low-sodium tomato juice, and I like to drink this during the ON day to keep up with my potassium and magnesium intake, while not loading up on salt.

Breaking OFF day rules: When to reset the ON/OFF schedule.

Because of social situations, you may need to go to a picnic or have a sit down dinner during an OFF day. This probably will hap-pen at least several times a month. Then the question is, should the next day be an OFF day, which would reset your schedule, or, should you go to another ON day, which means staying on your current schedule? What you should do depends on how much food you took in during the broken OFF day. The rule is this: At the end of a broken OFF day, if you have still managed to limit your intake to 800 calories, then you can stay on schedule and keep the next day as an ON day. If, on the other hand, you really did eat a lot of food (e.g., more than 800 calories worth) during a broken OFF day, it is better to reboot and change the next day into an OFF day.

If you find QOD eating just too strict for you

If you find your OFF days too hard to deal with, before abandoning QOD altogether, you might consider raising the 400 OFF-day calorie limit to 500 calories, especially if you combine QOD eating with a regular program of exercise. You will have to watch your calories a bit more during your ON day; your scale will tell you if the diet is working or not. If you are losing less than 4 lbs per month, then QOD eating is not working like it's supposed to. There are many other diets and surely there is one out there for you.

CHAPTER 8

THE IMPORTANCE OF EXERCISE

E XERCISE has unquestioned value in weight loss. And we'll definitely focus here on what exercise can do for you in helping you shed pounds. But after we've taken a look at how exercise contributes to weight loss, we'll also take a holistic view of exercise, noting its value in ways not directly related to weight loss. Most health experts and associations—including the American College of Sports Medicine, the National Institutes of Health, the Centers for Disease Control and Prevention, and the American Heart Association—recommend 30 minutes of moderate exercise at least five days a week as a minimum for reaping health benefits.[1]

How exercise can help in weight loss

Dieting alone *can* help you lose weight. Since 3,500 calories equals one pound of fat, you should, in theory, lose about a pound a week simply by cutting 500 calories a day from your diet. This does not quite happen because your calorie burn rate goes down with ordinary fasting, but this is another story. Another way to lose weight is to burn more calories. If you burn 500 additional calories a day through exercise, you should theoretically lose about a pound a week. So weight loss is a matter of balance. If your daily energy intake equals your total burn rate, you maintain your weight. If you take in more than you burn, you gain weight. And if you burn more than you take in, your weight goes down.

While it is possible to lose weight by cutting down on your total daily caloric intake, a growing body of research suggests that those who *keep the weight off* are those who combine dietary changes with regular exercise. "The No. 1 predictor of long-term success in essentially every weight maintenance study ever published is regular physical activity," says John P. Foreyt, Ph.D., director of the Nutrition Research Clinic at Baylor College of Medicine, Houston.[2]

According to the American Council on Exercise, there are three keys to a good exercise program: aerobics, strength training, and flexibility and core muscle training.[3]

Aerobic, strength and flexibility exercises and eating QOD

You can and should exercise while you are eating QOD. Until you see how your body adjusts to QOD eating, you may want to stick to low intensity and flexibility exercises at first, especially during your OFF day and on the morning of your ON day. However, I've found that one can often tolerate some aerobic exercise during the OFF day. Make sure that you always drink enough water, and keep up your sodium intake according to the guidelines given in this book. If your exercise does cause you to sweat a lot, you may need to drink more water to stay comfortable.

At least initially, don't exercise on the morning of your ON day, especially if you don't feel 100%, and always wait at least 1 hour after eating before attempting aerobic or any other more strenuous

---

To lose weight you can:

- Cut the number of calories in
- Increase the number of calories burned
- Do both (this is best of all!)

exercise. You may find yourself hungry after exercising—if so, you should eat what your body is directing you toward eating.

Let's take a look at how each of these types of exercise can help you not only reach your weight-loss goals, but maintain your new weight permanently.

Aerobics

Also called cardiovascular exercise—or in the health club lingo, simply "cardio." This form of exercise first received its name and came to national—and ultimately worldwide—attention in 1968, with the publication of a groundbreaking book by Kenneth Cooper titled *Aerobics*.[4] In his book, Dr. Cooper stresses the importance of physical activity that involves or improves the body's consumption of oxygen. Aerobic exercise is defined as any activity that uses the body's large muscle groups, can be maintained for a long period of time, and is rhythmic in nature. Aerobic exercise trains the heart, lungs, and cardiovascular system to process and deliver oxygen more quickly and efficiently to all parts of the body. The heart muscle becomes stronger and more efficient, pumping a larger volume of blood with each stroke. This means that fewer strokes are required to more rapidly transport oxygen throughout the body. Someone who becomes aerobically fit can work longer and harder, yet recover more quickly at the end of aerobic activity.

To be considered aerobic, an activity must be performed at a level of effort that causes your heart rate and breathing to increase.

One chart for determining your target heart rate is the following from the National Heart, Lung and Blood Institute.[5]

Age	Target Heart Rate Zone
25 years	98–146 beats per minute
35 years	93–138 beats per minute
45 years	88–131 beats per minute
55 years	83–123 beats per minute
65 years	78–116 beats per minute

Your goal should be to exercise at an intensity that keeps your heart rate in its "target" zone for at least 20 minutes.

Perhaps the chief benefit of aerobic exercise for weight loss is its help in burning fat. Depending on one's weight, such aerobic activities as running, walking, or swimming can burn a gratifying number of calories. As an example, someone weighing 150 pounds who walks at the rate of three miles per hour for one hour burns 320 calories. Increase the speed to a slow run of 5.5 miles per at same hour results in 660 calories burned. One additional bonus of aerobic exercise: Even after you finish exercising, your body continues to burn calories at an elevated rate for several more hours.

Strength training

For many years, aerobic exercise was thought to be the activity of choice for losing weight and keeping it off. But in recent years, renewed attention and research has focused on the advantages of strength training—also called *resistance training* or *weight training*—in contributing to weight loss.

The primary contribution of weight training to weight loss is that it builds new muscle tissue. Muscle tissue is highly active metabolically—each pound of muscle burns up to 35 calories a day even at rest. And of course, during the time your muscles are being challenged by exercise, muscles burn even more. Strength training also elevates the rate at which you burn calories for hours after you complete your exercise, so-called "metabolic afterburn." "Strength training ... produces a large increase in metabolic rate during the exercise session, a moderate increase in metabolic rate during the postexercise recovery period, and a small increase in resting metabolism throughout the day."[6]—says exercise physiologist Wayne Westcott, author of such books as *Building Strength and Stamina* and *Strength Training Past 50*.

Researchers at Tufts University studied older men and women who performed 30 minutes of strength training exercises three days a week for 12 weeks. Over the course of the study, these men and women added an average of three pounds of muscle and lost four pounds of fat. Yet to maintain their starting body weight, they had to eat 370 more calories a day—a 15 percent increase in their daily intake. The three pounds of new muscle elevated their resting metabolic rate by an average of 7 percent.[7]

You should not expect to build muscle using strength training during the period of QOD dieting, since your goal is to lose weight. But you should still do this to help preserve and tone the muscles that you have.

Abdominal muscle strengthening and flexibility training

The Pilates method[8] of strengthening muscles in the abdomen, along your spine, and around your hip joints has recently become popular. Pilates exercises will cause you to burn additional calories, and they also will improve the way you look, especially in the abdominal area. Increasing the strength of the core muscles around your spine will improve your posture and increase your flexibility.

Especially as we get older, our muscles and joints aren't as flexible as they once were. Even conditioned athletes can pay a price if they don't take time to properly warm up and cool down. Flexibility exercises help us become not just strong, but toned and supple. They can improve posture and breathing and help us move more gracefully. In addition, flexibility exercises seem to have a calming, centering effect on our minds and emotions. Practitioners of such ancient exercise forms as yoga have long known this.

Less intense exercise: Walking, slow swimming or water walking, and movements in the course of daily activities

Not everyone wants to jog or run marathons. Some find that brisk walking suits them better. Let me share a bit of my personal preference at this point. I have discovered that instead of compartmentalizing my life so that my "work" and "exercise" are separate, I can combine them so I'm doing both at the same time!

At home, I have set up an entire "mini-office" so that I can work on the computer, make phone calls, take care of paperwork—all while walking on my treadmill at a slow, comfortable 1.5 miles per hour or so. To accomplish this, I've had to create a stable platform—a "desk," if you will—on which I place my notebook computer, my phone, and other items. Since the platform is anchored to a wall and is not connected in any way to the treadmill, there's no vibration. In this way, I can spend several hours at a time doing my work while steadily burning calories. For those interested, you can see the details of my setup by clicking on the following link: *eatQOD.com/treadmill/treadmill.htm.*

Slow swimming is another great exercise. It is particularly useful because you can start slowly and proceed at your own pace. Even walking in the pool against the resistance of water is very useful, and will help bring your body into better shape as well as burn additional calories.

Burning calories during normal activity: Perhaps you're not yet ready to commit to a formal exercise plan. If you're not inclined toward the more common forms of exercise, you should know that carrying out ordinary activities can burn calories and improve your health:

Consider these ways that a 140-pound person can burn off 100 calories:

Activity	Minutes
Clean/vacuum/mop	25–35
Wash dishes	45–50
Wash windows	20–30
Rake leaves	20–25
Gardening	15–20
Shovel snow	10–15
Wax car	15–20
Stack firewood	15–20
Mow lawn	25–30

Source: Medical College of Wisconsin[9]

To burn more calories each day, deliberately commit to becoming more active. Take the stairs, not the elevator. Park way out at the end of the lot and walk to the store from there. Instead of "vegging out" on the couch in front of the TV, grab a glove and play catch with the kids. Take a walk around the block every night after supper.

Interestingly, people who "fidget" a lot burn extra calories each day with all this extra movement. I'm not suggesting you load up on espresso so you shake and shimmy all day—the point here is that lots of small movements can add up to an impressive amount of energy burned.

Benefits beyond weight loss

Exercise contributes not just to physical health, but also to mental, emotional, social, and even spiritual health. Many health organizations acknowledge the contribution of regular exercise to our overall health—to the health and improved life of the *whole person.*

So whether or not you choose to exercise in order to lose weight, I want to strongly encourage you—if you haven't already done so—to begin a program of daily exercise that fits your lifestyle and personality.

If you haven't been exercising, you may consider having your physician or primary health professional evaluate you first, to be sure there are no conditions that would affect your decision to exercise. It's always a good idea to get professional advice and even occasional monitoring as you engage in a program of increased physical exercise. Consider your doctor or primary health care provider to be a valued and knowledgeable partner in your efforts toward better health.

It's said that design implies function. That means that you can deduce what something is supposed to do by examining how it's made. And everything about the human body says that it's made to move. We're designed for action. You and I were not made to be couch potatoes. So, dear reader, please put down this book. Stand up. Walk around. Get those muscles moving. Pull some air into those lungs. Do it—and do it now!

The American Heart Association lists the following benefits of consistent daily exercise:[10]

- Reduces the risk of heart disease by improving blood circulation throughout the body

- Keeps weight under control

- Improves blood cholesterol levels

- Prevents and manages high blood pressure

- Prevents bone loss

- Boosts energy level

- Helps manage stress

- Releases tension

- Improves the ability to fall asleep quickly and sleep well

- Improves self-image

- Counters anxiety and depression and increases enthusiasm and optimism

- Increases muscle strength, increasing the ability to do other physical activities

- Provides a way to share an activity with family and friends

- Establishes good heart-healthy habits in children and counters the conditions (obesity, high blood pressure, poor cholesterol levels, poor lifestyle habits, etc.) that lead to heart attack and stroke later in life

- In older people, helps delay or prevent chronic illnesses and diseases associated with aging and maintains quality of life and independence longer

CHAPTER 9

CLARIFYING THE MIND AND SPIRIT

W HILE IT'S TRUE that QOD will help you lose weight, this approach to eating has other potential benefits to offer, including those that affect the broader person.

You and I—all of us—are more than just bodies. We're a complex blend of the physical, mental, emotional, social, and spiritual. Because of this, an entire school of medical thought has emerged in recent decades known as *holistic* medicine. Holistic medicine believes in addressing people not just as bodies in need of fixing, but as *whole* human beings. When something goes wrong in one's body, it's sometimes difficult to address the problem without also inquiring into the possible *non*physical causes behind it. The body, mind, spirit—indeed, all that make us fully human—are intricately related. So what affects one "part" of us can have definite consequences for the "rest" of us. The intimate connection between the mind and body has been demonstrated by an abundance of scientific inquiry.

In this chapter we will be exploring the mental and spiritual dimensions of fasting. Now, whether you personally view the spiritual as a relationship with a divine being or instead, a focus on what

lies beyond the immediate and tangible, this chapter can be of benefit. Some of you may also want to explore and experience the more
spiritual benefits that brief periods of fasting can bring your way.

If you are highly skeptical of the religious and spiritual, the purpose of this chapter is not to accomplish any major shift in your
thinking. And if your belief system includes the religious, neither is it
the purpose of this chapter to present the QOD diet in chiefly religious terms.

It's a fact, however, that fasting is most strongly linked to religious faith and practice. And though this is not a primary focus of
the QOD diet, there are benefits of this plan that can best be under-
stood in the context of how fasting is practiced in various religious
traditions.

Judaism

In the Jewish tradition there are two major and five minor fast
days. By far the most important is Yom Kippur—or "Day of
Atonement"—the holiest day of the Jewish year. This day typically
occurs in October.[1] The Yom Kippur fast is observed for a 25-hour
period, beginning at sunset on one day and extending past sunset the
next. It is observed eight days following Rosh Hashana, the Jewish
New Year. Yom Kippur is a time for introspection, self-correction,
prayer, and repentance.

Christianity

Lent is a forty-day period prior to Easter. Ash Wednesday, the
day after "fat Tuesday," or "Mardi gras," is the day that Catholics
begin their Lenten fast. During Lent, Catholics forego meat on
Fridays. Also, by tradition, they give up a favorite food—say chocolate or beer—for the entire Lenten period. On Ash Wednesday and
Good Friday, the Friday just before Easter, Catholics are supposed
to eat only once during the day.[2]

Catholics are not the only Christians who fast. Fasting reaches
back to the earliest years of the Christian church. According to Biblical

accounts, Jesus Christ himself fasted for forty days at the beginning of his ministry. So too did the prophet John the Baptist. No record exists, however, that Christ ever commanded or expected those who believed in him to follow his example in fasting. Nonetheless, instances of fasting—usually coupled with prayer—are noted in the New Testament, and Christians from the beginning have followed the example of their Old Testament spiritual ancestors in fasting.

Protestant Christians do not fast in observance of any particular religious days. Nor is fasting generally presented as a requirement. But Protestants do fast both individually and as groups in order to heighten spiritual sensitivity so as to better connect with God, to demonstrate repentance for sin, or to focus requests presented in prayer. Groups of Christians sometimes fast in pursuit of spiritual renewal and revival.

Buddhism

All of the main branches of Buddhism practice some periods of fasting, typically on full-moon days and other holidays. Buddha himself, having concluded from his own experience that mortification or punishment of the body does not lead to enlightenment, proposed a less-extreme form of fasting. Therefore Buddhist monks are permitted to eat most anything, but in moderation.[3] Buddha advised monks not

---

Spiritual reasons for which people have fasted throughout the ages:
- To atone for sins and demonstrate repentance
- Spiritual self-purification
- As discipline for the body
- To clear the mind and spirit for communion with God
- As preparation for an important religious ceremony
- To quiet the body so as to listen to the mind and soul
- To demonstrate intensity and sincerity in prayer requests
- As an adjunct to mourning
- As preparation to cast out devils or diseases

to take solid food after noon. Lay Buddhists who observe the Eight Precepts of Buddhism also abstain from eating solid food after noon on full-moon days.

For the Buddhist, brief fasting is believed to cleanse both body and spirit and is seen as helping to achieve spiritual enlightenment. This is to be a time of heightened awareness and concentration on the essential in regard to such concerns as language, behavior, clothing, place, and food. It is to be a time devoted to much pray   -tation. Fasting is seen as a means of freeing the mind and as an exercise in self-control and self-discipline.

Islam

Fasting is one of the Five Pillars (duties) of Islam. Muslim belief is that during the month of Ramadan[4]—the ninth month of the Islamic year—Allah revealed the first verses of Islam's holy book, the Koran, to the Prophet Muhammad.

The prophet is to have said: "Ramadan is the month during which the Koran was revealed, providing guidance for the people, clear teachings, and the Statute Book. Those of you who witness this month shall fast therein."[5]

The Islamic Ramadan fast includes complete abstinence for the month from foods, drinks, marital relations, and smoking. This harsh requirement becomes possible because the period of fasting begins each day at dawn but ends at sunset.

Ramadan is a time of intensive worship, reading of the Koran, purifying one's behavior, and doing such good deeds as giving to charity. As with some of the other religious traditions already noted, the Ramadan fast is also intended as an opportunity to practice self-control and to cleanse body and mind. As they experience daily hunger and thirst, Muslims are to be reminded of the suffering of the poor and chronically hungry.

Before leaving this glimpse of fasting as practiced in Islam, I want to share a brief conversation said to have occurred between one "Abdullah Ibn Amr" and the Prophet Muhammad. You'll notice an interesting similarity to the eating pattern of the QOD diet!

As presented, the conversation was to have proceeded as follows: [6]

Abdullah: "I have strength to fast."

The Prophet: "Observe the fast of David, no more."

Abdullah: "What is it?"

The Prophet: "Half the *dahr* [time]" "Fast one day and break the fast another."

Abdullah: "But I can do better."

The Prophet: "There ... better."

On another occasion, the Prophet is said to have said "Abdullah, I was told that you spend the day fasting and the night in prayer." Abdullah answered in the affirmative, whereupon the Prophet commanded him with these words: "Do not do so. Fast one day and break it the next. Pray part of the night and sleep the rest. You have an obligation toward your body, your eyes, and your wife."

The Prophet's reference to the "fast of David" is undoubtedly to the record of Islamic history that holds: "The most beloved fasting to Allah was the fasting of the Prophet David, who used to fast alternate days."

Whatever the Prophet's reasons for advocating the every-other-day fast, it goes to show that the idea of alternating fasting days with days of eating has been around for more than a thousand years.

Hinduism

Fasting in Hinduism is an exercise in denial of the physical needs and sensory desires of the body for the sake of spiritual gain. According to the Hindu scriptures, fasting assists in bringing about a harmony between body and soul. This is seen as vital to human well-being, as it nourishes both physical and spiritual demands. [7]

As Hindus see it, the demands of daily life and distracting physical indulgences combine to make concentration on the spiritual difficult. Worshipers must therefore strive to impose restraints on themselves in order to focus the mind on spiritual things. One such form of restraint is fasting.

Hindu fasting can involve anything ranging from a strict twenty-four-hour abstinence from all food and drink, to foregoing specific food items such as salt or cereals.

The underlying principle behind Hindu fasting is found in *Ayurveda*[8]—the ancient Indian system of medicine. This philosophy holds that the cause of many diseases is the accumulation of toxins in the digestive system. By fasting, the digestive organs are rested, and the body is cleansed and balanced.

Mormonism

Mormons are instructed to fast the first Sunday of each month.[9] Individuals, families, or even entire wards (a ward is a territorial division of a Mormon settlement) may engage in such fasts as they choose. On the first-Sunday fast, Mormons forego food and drink for two consecutive meals. The money and/or food they save is donated to the needy. Following the fast, members participate in a "fast and testimony meeting."

Among the intended goals of Mormon fasting is achieving closeness to God, or perhaps as an adjunct to a petition to God for healing or assistance with a difficult decision.

How this may apply to QOD fasting

So religious reasons for fasting are many and varied. Many of these reasons might apply to the alternate days of near-fasting that are a part of QOD. Your personal religious convictions or spiritual interest may dictate which of these reasons you find worth including in your own fasting experience. But even if you are not particularly religious—or even if you are nonreligious—there are benefits to brief periods of fasting that can be yours. And these benefits will exist regardless of whether you choose to see them in a religious or spiritual context.

We often are so consumed with the fast-track pursuits of our daily life that we rarely if ever take time to pull back and get perspective—a view of the larger picture. Choosing to alternate days of normal eating with days of fasting gives both body and mind a chance to break the habitual—the activities that have become so automatic, that we do them without conscious thought.

Have you ever thought of what music would be like if it had no silent spaces between the notes? It's the alternating bands of sound and silence that give music its beauty and power. In the same way, you and I were not meant to be always ON—always going and doing and eating. We need to build into our eating deliberate times of silence—of being OFF instead of ON.

Have you ever blasted the radio for hours on a long road trip? If so, have you ever turned the radio off, only to notice for the first time the reassuring hum of your car's motor? Fasting is like turning down the radio. When we do, we can hear other sounds. The sound of our own body, letting us know what it wants and needs. The sound of our uninterrupted thoughts, bringing us insights, solutions, perspectives.

Ironically, "fasting" is in a very real sense "slowing." Slowing down to listen. Slowing down long enough to think, to contemplate, to meditate, to pursue the greater truths and realities outside of ourselves.

No, you don't need to endanger your health by fasting for long periods of time. The whole idea of fasting is to achieve some balance in your life—and a long fast creates imbalance. The idea of fasting is to bring very real, experiential benefits to yourself. And this can be well achieved through brief fasts of just one day, alternating with days when you eat as you normally do. It's opening yourself to "something more." And it's yours to be found in QOD!

HEALTH AND LONGEVITY
ADDING LIFE TO YOUR YEARS—AND
YEARS TO YOUR LIFE

L et's get one thing straight at the outset. At this time, there is no proven health benefit in humans of eating every other day. The research required to prove this would be difficult and time-consuming, and just has not been done. However, there is intriguing evidence from both animal and short-term human studies that reducing the amount of food we eat might not only improve our health but may add years to our lives.

Over recent decades, human *life expectancy* has increased dramatically. In 1930, life expectancy for men was 58 years—and for women, just under 62. By 2001, these figures had risen to over 74 for men and just under 80 for women. Improved health care, vaccinations, and higher living standards each contributed, undoubtedly, to this improved life expectancy.

But there's a difference between *life expectancy* and *maximum human lifespan*. It's still considered remarkable when someone reaches 100 years of age. Typically, the oldest people in the world die off between 110 and 120 years of age. But some scientists who specialize in life extension studies are convinced that it's possible that human beings could routinely live to 120 or beyond, with just one change to diet alone. That change is *caloric restriction*, and the results of studies in rodents, fish, insects, and even primates have promising implications for human lifespan as well.

The connection between eating less and living longer first emerged in the 1930s when a Cornell University nutrition professor—the late Clive McCay and his colleagues unexpectedly found that rats fed a calorically-restricted diet lived up to 30 percent longer.[1]

According to Luigi Fontana, a geriatrics researcher at Washington University in St. Louis, the shortage of food in some northern European countries during the two world wars led to a dramatic decrease in mortality rates from coronary heart disease, type 2 diabetes, and cancer. He noted that after the wars, the rates surged again.[2] It's also been noted that people on the Japanese island of Okinawa, where residents have long followed a calorically restricted diet, have the longest average lifespan in the world as well as the highest documented percentage of centenarians. Okinawans eat 40 percent fewer calories than do Americans.[3]

A number of studies are currently in process to determine the effects of caloric restriction on monkeys. The University of Wisconsin, the University of Maryland, and the National Institute on Aging (NIA) are among the entities currently conducting such research.

Perhaps one of the best-known researchers in the area of life extension is Roy Walford, Professor of Pathology at the University of California at Los Angeles. For decades, Dr. Walford has been a leading researcher in the effects of caloric restriction on a variety of laboratory animals. In his laboratory at the UCLA Medical Center, for example, he has demonstrated that caloric restriction results in a very substantial extension in the lifespan of fish. By applying systematic underfeeding, he has achieved similar results in mice, rats, house-pets, and even some microscopic forms of life.[4]

Such laboratory animals, says Susan Roberts, Senior Scientist and Director of the Energy Metabolism Laboratory at Tufts University, "don't just live longer, they are healthier. They age more slowly. Their hair has gone gray less quickly. Their hormones have stayed at their youthful profile, and their immune function has stayed good."[5]

Skeptics will point out—and have—that people aren't lab mice, and that results of rodent research don't automatically apply to humans. Aware of this, Dr. Walford decided to test some of these concepts in humans. He and seven other researchers, four men and four women, spent two years, from 1991 to 1993, in a closed ecological environment called Biosphere 2, near Oracle, Arizona. During their stay in the Biosphere, Walford and his colleagues practiced a carefully monitored regimen of caloric restriction, similar to that used in his laboratory animals. At the conclusion of this 2-year period, Dr. Walford found clear-cut evidence that the same physiological changes that had occurred in rodents on calorie-restricted diets also took place in human beings.[6] Might the same calorie-restricted diets that lengthened lifespan in laboratory animals prolong life in humans? The Biosphere experiment lasted only two years. Dr. Walford believes that a time could come when human beings too might alter their diets over an entire lifetime, with a similar dramatic extension of lifespan.

One of the biggest criticisms of the idea of caloric restriction as a method of extending life is that a lifetime of dieting would result in perpetual hunger. Dr. Walford counters by pointing out that if we change the quality of what we eat—consuming what he calls "nutrient-dense" food instead of the typical American junk-food diet—we will be satisfied even when eating fewer calories. He calls this dietary approach "undernutrition without malnutrition."[7] Somehow, though, the prospect of a lifetime of restricted caloric intake doesn't seem all that appealing.

Some recently published research indicates that it might be possible to obtain the health benefits of a calorically restricted diet—*without actually having to go on one!* In 2003, research completed at the National Institute on Aging was reported in the *Proceedings of the National Academy of Sciences*. Lead researcher Mark Mattson conducted research on mice that not only supports the conclusions of Dr. Walford and others—it also supports the potential of the QOD diet! Dr. Mattson and his colleagues found that mice fed *every other day* (sound familiar?) but allowed to eat all they wanted on the days they did eat, enjoyed the same health benefits—including lower blood sugar and more stress tolerance—as mice that ate every day but had their calories reduced by 40 percent.[8] Let's make one thing clear: this study did not measure lifespan—only blood levels of various key mediators linked to stress and shortened lifespan, but these results were remarkable, nevertheless.

Now, obviously, the reason I'm advocating the QOD diet in this book is for its short-term use to assist in losing weight. Still, results such as these suggest that perhaps a modified, longer-term plan of QOD eating may be an inherently gentler and more bioc̶e̶ ̶̶ way of taking in our food.

Why is reducing calories so beneficial to our health? Researchers theorize that a reduced caloric intake protects cells throughout the body; they die more slowly and repair themselves more easily. Some scientists believe that, like hibernation, restricting calories significantly slows the physical processes that cause wear and tear on the body. When cells convert food to energy, they release byproducts called *free radicals*. These biochemical villains inflict damage on cells, tissues, and genes—and have been implicated in age-related changes ranging from facial wrinkles to increased cancer risk. Cutting calories reduces the quantity of these harmful free radicals.[9]

"We think what happens," says NIA's Dr. Mattson, "is that going without food imposes a mild stress on cells, and cells respond by increasing their ability to cope with more severe stress. It's sort of analogous to physical effects of exercise on muscle cells."[10] For example, evidence from Dr. Mattson's research shows that caloric restriction protects mouse brain cells from developing such diseases as Alzheimer's and Parkinson's.[11]

"Whatever the underlying process," says Thomas Perls, a Harvard Medical School Professor and author of the book *Living to 100*—"it does appear that caloric restriction is an important mechanism of slowing down the aging process."[12]

Whether or not it's accompanied by caloric restriction, the QOD diet appears to have some encouraging and solid science supporting the idea that every-other-day eating can potentially benefit one's overall health. Lifespan? It's too early to tell in people, and I am not advocating staying on the QOD diet for more than 4–6 months at a time. But just possibly, less may be more.

CHAPTER 11

TEN REASONS TO GET STARTED

If you're willing to be dedicated and disciplined enough to follow the program, the QOD diet will work for you. Here are 10 reasons to try it:

1. You can lose a significant amount of weight, yet not feel starved.

This might seem impossible for an eating plan that relies on restricting food intake every other day. But if you follow the plan outlined in this book, you can do exactly what's needed to keep your body from feeling hungry and weak.

2. You're never more than a day away from "normal" eating.

With QOD eating you know that the very next day, you can have complete, satisfying meals again.

3. QOD prevents your body's starvation alarms from going off.

Our bodies are designed so that after two or three consecutive days of significant caloric restriction, metabolism—the rate at which food is burned for energy—is markedly reduced. On QOD, you lower calorie intake for only one day—not long enough to trigger the body's starvation response.

4. QOD puts you in touch with those foods that your body really needs.

By letting the body rest every other day, you discover, perhaps for the first time ever, that you can *"hear" your body "talking" to* letting you know what sort of foods your body needs and wants.

5. Your food will taste better.

I don't know why this happens, but it does. When eating QOD you'll make a wonderful discovery. You will find that you have become sensitized to the rich flavors of the foods you eat, and to their nuances of taste, texture, and aroma.

6. QOD helps you break the cycle of "mindless eating."

We often eat *reactively* instead of *proactively*. On QOD, you learn how to *take the initiative in making food choices*.

7. QOD gives your body a regular, much-needed rest.

People who are constantly eating never give their digestive system or their kidneys a rest. QOD gives your body a chance to maintain, repair, and tune itself up.

8. QOD may well contribute to a healthier life, and just maybe, to a longer one.

Although there is no direct evidence of a QOD health benefit for people at this time, regular caloric restriction has been shown to improve health and perhaps extend our lifespan.

9. QOD can help clarify your mind and spirit.

Many people have found new insights, a new understanding of life and their place in it, and even a new awareness of something beyond themselves, by eating less food or by fasting.

10. The emphasis of QOD is on balance and moderation in your life.

On QOD, you eat a balance of fats, protein, and carbohydrates. You combine a sensible program of exercise with your changed way of eating in order to lose weight and to keep it off.

CHAPTER 12

YOU'VE REACHED YOUR TARGET WEIGHT —NOW WHAT?

G rowing up, we absorbed the practical wisdom of our parents, teachers, and others who learned by personal experience several important rules of life:

"Anything worth having takes work."

"If something sounds too good to be true, it probably is."

"There's no such thing as something for nothing."

Yet despite all this hard-won, proven wisdom, you can't live a day without somebody offering an easy way of getting what you want without paying any price. No work. No effort. No sacrifice. And when it comes to hype, hooey, and flat-out lies, the purveyors of weight-loss promises take a back seat to no one. Wanna lose? Take our pill, and you don't need to change what or how much you eat— the fat will just melt off. Try our plan, and even without exercise, you'll lose 20 pounds in a month.

It's bunk—and you know it.

So instead, you've chosen a sound, steady way to lose weight— perhaps the QOD diet—and you've arrived now at your target weight. But you didn't get here without some commitment, some effort, some discipline, and some sacrifice. Arriving at your goal weight was a day of well-deserved pride and exhilaration.

But as most of us already know, losing weight is not the hardest part of the challenge. It's maintaining the new weight afterward. Millions of people diet each year. Many of them achieve their goal. But the sad statistical truth is that, even with the best diets, after 5 years, most people gain back more than ¾ of the weight that they had initially lost[1]. Some dieters even end up weighing more than when they started.

I don't want that to happen to you. So I'm going to repeat here another of those common sense bits of wisdom: *"If you keep doing what you always did, you'll keep getting what you always got."*

When you arrive at your goal, it's decision time: You can decide to throw off all restrictions and return to your old way of eating—the way that made you fat—or—you can choose a new way of eating. A way that's less restrictive than your diet, but different than the way you once ate. Your new way of eating should be one that you can comfortably live with—yet one that will help you to maintain your new weight. Here are several suggestions:

Periodically, dust off QOD and use it again briefly

Perhaps my first suggestion could be summarized in another old saying: *"Dance with the one that brung ya."* If QOD got you to your goal, then every now and then, QOD can get you back on track if you drift a little.

After your weight-loss effort is ended, you're still going to have times when, for any number of reasons, you find yourself "falling off the wagon"—slipping back into old eating patterns. Maybe it's a holiday time, and the house is suddenly full of pies and cookies and pastries and sweets. You end up eating way too much food and carbs and find yourself entering a vicious cycle of cravings that require ever more carbs to satisfy.

If this happens, it may be time to "dance" with QOD again. Not for months or weeks. Just a short spin around the floor for a week or so. Having "done" QOD, you have learned to "hear" your body—and by now you'll know when your body is on a carb-craving bender and when it's not.

So go right back to how you ate while you were losing. Alternate those ON and OFF days. Cut way back on carbs—especially the highly processed, sugar-laden kind that create cravings. Be sure to get enough protein and healthy fats. Keep your OFF day calories under 300–400 a day. And in no time, you'll notice the carb-cravings are back under control.

Another good reason to keep QOD close at hand is that even if you don't get yourself into a carb-craving trap, you may occasionally simply eat too much. Despite all the best intentions, it can be a tall order to avoid overeating at Thanksgiving—or when you go out to a restaurant that serves mountains of irresistible food. You can follow up such days with a few days of eating QOD, and you're back on track again.

One of the really good things that QOD did for you originally was to help you make conscious food choices based on what your body was telling you. If you get to the place where you're not really in the driver's seat anymore—you're eating in response to visual or other stimuli around you—it's time to reclaim control over your eating choices. A brief return to QOD will help that happen.

Eating QOD for short periods can also "reset" both the body and the mind. You may find that at times, you're eating too often, are nervous, can't concentrate or focus—you just can't get any productive work done. You need a chance to settle down, clear your mind, and become more "aware" again, not only of what you're eating but of who you are.

Finally, you can return to QOD if you find your weight creeping up. Daily weight fluctuations are normal for anyone, but if you find that your weight has increased so that it's consistently 5 or more pounds above your goal weight, it may be time to go back to dieting for a brief time. It's far easier to eat QOD for a month to lose 5 pounds than to let yourself get 25 pounds overweight, at which point you will need to eat QOD for 4–6 months to lose your excess weight.

So in summary, shorter periods of QOD dieting can be a valuable tool to put you back in touch with what your body really needs and wants. QOD can help you break bad eating habits before they get out of control. It can clear you mind. QOD can keep you close to your best weight. Returning to use QOD for short periods is much like rebooting your computer. Just restart and move ahead again.

Stock your living space with an abundance of the right foods

Another great help in maintaining your new weight is to be sure of two things: that you have stripped your home (and office too, for that matter) of all the wrong kinds of food—the ones that you know put on the pounds—and that you have stocked your place with a broad choice of the right kinds of foods.

Already in this book, we've touched on the kinds of foods that help you not just lose weight, but maintain it. Be sure you have plenty of complex carbs like fruit, veggies, and whole grains around. Read your food labels and stay away from anything loaded with sugar and/or saturated fat. Keep at hand a variety of foods to snack on: baby carrots, celery strips, nonfat or low-fat yogurt, nuts (I personally find a handful of walnuts to be a great snack), some raisins, some low-fat string cheese sticks. Tomato-vegetable juice is always nice to have around when you're really hungry for a bit of salt, and orange juice is a great way to get the carb boost that you sometimes need.

And remember some of the other guidelines you've learned about earlier in the book: as you deliberately limit certain kinds of carbs, don't offset this by overloading on protein. And don't be afraid of fats—your body not only needs the right kinds of fats, but some fats can actually help keep your arteries clear and your weight under control. Oils high in unsaturated fats, such as canola, soybean, and safflower, and especially olive oil—are good for cooking or on salads. And some oils, such as flaxseed oil, contain high levels of essential omega fatty acids that fight cholesterol and assist with fat burning. Nuts, olives, and avocados too, all contain good fats that contribute to good health.

Control your portion sizes

As you approach your goal weight, you can't escape the choice you must make. You can choose to "finish" your diet and return to eating the same portion sizes as you did before—or you can decide to deliberately, consciously downsize your portions. And here we return to this matter of desserts, sweets, and other such calorie-rich foods that can so easily trigger carb cravings. Must you do without all such foods till the day you die? Absolutely not. But remember again that part of the reason you became overweight in the first place was that you didn't or couldn't control your intake of such foods. To stay at your ideal weight, you have no ch: scipline yourself to relate to your "trigger" foods in a whole new way. Go ahead and have a piece of pie or cake—but make it a thin slice, and eat it slowly, savoring every morsel. If someone gives you a box of chocolates, ration them out to yourself at the rate of one every other day or so. If you have ice cream, don't eat from the carton—get a small dessert dish and have a scoop or two. The refrigerator will keep the rest till later, just fine.

Combine changed eating habits with exercise

In a previous chapter we discussed the importance of exercise for weight loss. Exercise boosts metabolism so you burn more calories. Also, exercise builds new muscle tissue—which is very metabolically active; the more muscle you add, the more calories those added muscles burn.

Exercise also assists with digestion and elimination, helps stabilize blood glucose levels, and keeps your heart and arteries strong and clear of buildup. Add to these benefits the improvement exercise has on mood, sleep, and general outlook—and you don't want to do without it. So as part of your new way of living fit and trim, you'll find that exercise is indispensable. If you try rowing across a lake with one oar—and you row on just one side, you may eventually get where you're going, but it's going to take a long time and be very difficult. Get both of your oars—sensible eating, and regular exercise—into the water, and you'll never again need those amazingly large clothes you once wore.

In closing

If you pay attention to these suggestions, I have absolutely no doubt that you will maintain your new weight for the rest of your life.

CONGRATULATIONS!

I applaud your interest in changing your life for the better. Many things can motivate people to attempt losing weight. For some, it's to look better. For others, it's health concerns. Still others simply feel that they aren't in control of a major area of their lives. Most people have multiple reasons that drive them to change their lifestyle for the better.

Making the decision to change your weight takes initiative, courage, and determination. It shows that you care enough about yourself to put forth effort to improve. This says a lot of positive things about you.

I solidly support your decision and your efforts. I wish you success and the satisfaction of accomplishment. And for those of you who find QOD to be of help and value, I'd enjoy hearing from you.

We have included a feedback form at the back of this book. Please fill this out with your experiences and suggestions, and mail it back to our publisher or you can send suggestions and questions by email to *feedback@whiteswanbooks.com*.

— John T. Daugirdas, M.D.

BIBLIOGRAPHY, FOOTNOTES, AND RESOURCES

Foreword

1. **Uric acid and cardiovascular disease risk**
   Feig DI, Nakagawa T, Karumanchi SA, Oliver WJ, Kang DH, Finch J, Johnson RJ. Hypothesis: Uric acid, nephron number, and the pathogenesis of essential hypertension.
   Kidney Int. 2004 Jul;66(1):281–7.
   Comment: This is new information and is still controversial.

Chapter 2

1. **Binge eating and anorexia**
   National Institutes of Mental Health. Eating Disorders: Facts About Eating Disorders and the Search for Solutions. US. Gov't Printing Office, 2001.
   weblink: *nimh.nih.gov/publicat/eatingdisorders.cfm*

Comment: If you have any tendency to binge eating, QOD is not for you, and if you find yourself starting to binge eat while on QOD, stop the diet and don't look back.

2. Risk of heart attack with large meals

Lipovetzky N et al. Heavy meals as a trigger for a first event of the acute coronary syndrome: a case-crossover study.
Isr Med Assoc J. 2004 Dec;6(12):728–31.

Comment: There also was an abstract with similar findings presented to the American Heart Association in 2000 (by Lopez-Jimenez et al), but which is not yet published. For this reason, I don't recommend eating QOD for anyone who has had a heart attack, has had anginal type symptoms, or is otherwise at high risk of a heart attack. If you are following the QOD eating plan properly you should always eat 5–6 small meals during the ON day—but we are just excluding such people to play it extra safe.

3. Risk of postural hypotension after large meals

Puvi-Rajasingham S, Mathias CJ.
Effect of meal size on post-prandial blood pressure and on postural hypotension in primary autonomic failure.
Clin Auton Res. 1996 Apr;6(2):111–4.

Comment: This is a study in patients with an impaired nervous system, but postural hypotension is common in diabetics and also in the elderly, even without autonomic nervous system impairment. Postural hypotension may also be more common in people taking water pills or diuretics. For this reason, I do not recommend eating QOD for diabetics, people over 60, people who have had a stroke or near-stroke, people taking diuretics, or anyone who has had problems with low blood pressure or dizziness.

4. **Interaction of food with drug absorption and metabolism**

   Welling PG. Interactions affecting drug absorption.

   Clin Pharmacokinet. 1984 Sep-Oct;9(5):404–34.

   Comment: Food can affect not only absorption of drugs, but also metabolism of some drugs. If you are taking any prescription medication, always consult with your doctor before going on a QOD eating plan.

Chapter 3

1. **Obesity in the United States**

   Flegal KM, Graubard BI, Williamson DF, Gail MH. Excess deaths associated with underweight, overweight, and obesity.

   JAMA. 2005 Apr 20;293(15):1861–7.

2. **Influence of alternate day fasting on metabolic rate**

   Heilbronn LK et al. Alternate-day fasting in nonobese subjects: effects on body weight, body composition, and energy metabolism.

   Am J Clin Nutr. 2005 Jan;81(1):69–73.

   Comment: This was a short-term study in non-obese persons. Metabolic rate did not decrease over 22 days. The patients had a hard time not eating anything on their OFF days, however.

Chapter 4

1. **Biblical parable relating to house building**

   The reference is *Matthew 7:24–27*. The parable compares the stability of two houses, one built on sand, and one built on a rock. Matthew writes: "Therefore everyone who hears these words of mine and puts them into practice is like a wise man who built his house on the rock. The rain came down, the streams rose, and the winds blew and beat against that house; yet it did not fall, because it had its foundation on the rock. But everyone who hears these words of mine and does not put them into practice is like a foolish man who built his house on sand. The rain came down, the streams rose, and the winds blew and beat against that house, and it fell with a great crash."

2. Dietary guideline information

There are two good sites, one focusing on a set of recommendations sponsored by the Department of Agriculture in 20 which can be reached via *health.gov/dietaryguidelines/*, and the other based on the Institute of Medicine dietary recommendations, reachable via its website at *iom.edu*. Search for their Dietary Reference Intakes (DRIs): Recommended Intakes for Individuals, 2002. The current link (which can change), is: *iom.edu/ Object.File/Master/21/372/0.pdf*. Updated links will be available at *eatQOD.com*.

3. Importance of soft drinks as sources of added sugar

Guthrie JF, Morton JF. Food sources of added sweeteners in the diets of Americans.

J Am Diet Assoc. 2000 Jan;100(1):43–51

4. DASH diet

For more information on the DASH diet you can go to the following website: *dashdiet.org*.

5. Vitamin B12—oral supplementation in older people

Eussen SJ, de Groot LC, Clarke R, Schneede J, Ueland PM, Hoefnagels WH, van Staveren WA. Oral cyanocobalamin supplementation in older people with vitamin B-12 deficiency: a dose-finding trial.

Arch Intern Med. 2005 May 23;165(10):1167–72

Comment: The usual recommendation is that 3 micrograms per day of crystalline vitamin B-12 is enough, and that it should be taken by adults over 50 daily (see reference 2 above) but this recent paper suggests that 300 micrograms may be needed for some people. This only becomes an issue for people over 50 or who have some problem with vitamin B-12 absorption, although the amount of crystalline B-12 that vegans should take has not been well studied. The official recommendation, though is to take in only 3.0 micrograms per day.

6. Aristotle, Confucius, and ꞏ   ꞏean

As summarized by Dale Lugenbehl, in an essay written for Concepts in Ethics:

(teach.lanecc.edu/lugenbehld/201/handouts/Golden%20Mean.htm)

"Confucius was born around 550 BC in China and died in 479 BC. Confucius believed in living by what he called the "doctrine of the mean" or "golden mean" (chung yung or "constant middle"). For every action there are two extremes which must be avoided: the extreme of excess and the extreme of deficiency. What lies the proper distance between these extremes is virtue, and the right way to act. In a similar way in India, the Buddha (approximately 560–480 BC) taught that the right course is the "middle way."

Aristotle lived in Greece (384–322 BC). In his book Nicomachaean Ethics, he outlines what he also calls "the doctrine of the mean." What he has to say here is very similar in many ways to the views of Confucius, and he develops at length how this doctrine applies to determining what course of action is right in a number of different situations."

Chapter 5

1. Sodium intake 1500–2000 mg

The 2000 mg figure is OK for most people, but if you are African American or over 50, or if you can tolerate a lower sodium diet, the 1500 mg sodium OFF day goal is better, meets dietary guidelines, and probably is more healthful. 1500 mg should still work fine.

2. Dietary guideline information

See reference 2 in Chapter 4. Although the guidelines are for 4700 mg of potassium, it is impossible to eat that much on the OFF day without taking supplements, and I don't recommend this. Most Americans only eat about 2000 mg of potassium per day (on average) in any event. For calcium, the 800 mg OFF day target is lower than the recommended amount but should be sufficient for the OFF day.

3. High-bicarbonate mineral water

There is no evidence that drinking high-bicarbonate mineral water is bad, but there is a syndrome called milk-alkali, that causes problems if you take in too much bicarbonate and calcium together. On your OFF day you will be eating very little protein which is the main acid-generating food. Acid neutralizes bicarbonate. So with little dietary protein intake there is bit higher risk of winding up with more bicarbonate than you need. This is just my personal opinion. I believe that most mineral water brands, which usually contain a modest amount of bicarbonate, are fine to drink during the OFF day.

4. How much vitamin B-12 to take

See comments in reference 5, Chapter 4.

5. V-8™ vegetable juice, Kefir

The manufacturer of V-8 (Campbell Soup Company) and the manufacturer of Kwashenka/Kefir drinkable yogurt (Lifeway Foods) do not make any recommendations about using their products as part of a QOD eating plan.

Chapter 6

1. Calculating caloric intake during the ON day

How did we get to the ON day caloric target of 2000–2600 calories per day? In general, while following a diet you need to restrict average calories/day to 60% of your estimated maintenance daily energy intake. Maintenance means the amount of energy needed to keep a steady body weight.

If you go through the calculations, you find that a tall man who is normally active, when going on a diet would need to restrict food to about 1500 cal/day. Because energy requirement is less in women, and because energy requirement also depends on height, a short woman wo . o restrict intake to about 1200 cal/day while dieting. But that's for people eating every day. To get your goal calorie intake for your ON day you need to double these numbers to get how many calories you can eat over a 2-day period. Subtract your OFF day intake of 400, and what's left is the amount you can eat on your ON day. For example:

Tall (6' 0") man: 1500 x 2 = 3000. 3000 minus 400 = 2600
Small (5' 0") woman: 1200 x 2 = 2400. 2400 minus 400 = 2000

So ON day calorie goal for a tall man would be 2600 calories, while for a short woman the goal would be 2000 calories.

The estimated energy intake (the amount before you multiply by 60%) depends not only on gender and height, but also on age and, very much on a person's level of activity. The Harris-Benedict equation can be used to calculate the estimated energy expenditure for people of various sizes, ages, and activity levels. The formula is complicated but there are many websites out there that can crunch the numbers for you (see the links on *eatQOD.com*). You also can get this information from tables. One set of tables that I recommend is published by the Institute of Medicine and can be found at *iom.edu/Object.File/Master/21/372/0.pdf*. But again, this is only the first step. You have now found your estimated energy intake, but you still need to multiply this by 0.60 (60%), multiply again by 2, and subtract 400.

2. Food intake after a fast

Johnstone AM, et al., Effect of an acute fast on energy compensation and feeding behavior in lean men and women.

International Journal of Obesity and Related Metabolic Disorders, Dec. 2002, 26(12): 1623–1628.

3. Importance of breakfast
Schlundt DG, et al., The role of breakfast in the treatment of obesity: a randomized clinical trial.
Am J Clin Nutr. 1992, 55: 645–651.

Chapter 8

1. 30 minutes of moderate exercise per day
This recommendation is made by a number of health groups. The most well-known source of this recommendation was the US Surgeon General report in 1996. In September of 2002, the Institute of Medicine actually recommended doubling this amount. See: *US Department of Health and Human Services. The Surgeon General's call to action to prevent and decrease overweight and obesity.* Rockville, MD: US Department of Health and Human Services, Public Health Service, Office of the Surgeon General; 2001. (Available from US GPO, Washington)

2. Dr. John Foreyt citation
Interview with Dr. Foreyt on the Calories Count website, October 6, 2005. *health.caloriescount.com/isroot/caloriescount/SiteImages/ transcript_ drforeyt.html.*

3. American Council on Exercise citation
On the three components to a successful exercise program. See the page on their website (*Acefitness.org*) at this link: *acefitness.org/fitfacts/fitfacts_display.aspx?itemid=78.*

4. *Aerobics* by Kenneth Cooper
For a more recent book by the same author, see: *Aerobics* by Kenneth H. Cooper. Bantam. 1981. ISBN: 0553209922.

5. **Target Heart Rate**

This table is based on 50–75% of the expected maximum heart rate. A web reference to this data from the NHLBI can be found at this link: *pueblo.gsa.gov/cic_text/health/exercise-heart/page6.htm.*

6. **Wayne Westcott citations**

a. Wayne L. Westcott. *Builder and Stamina.* Human Kinetics Publishers, 2nd edition, January 2003. ISBN: 0736045155.

b. Wayne L. Westcott. Strength Training Past 50. Human Kinetics Publishers. October, 1997. ISBN: 0880117168.

7. **Campbell study**

Campbell W, Crim M, Young V, and Evans W. (1994). Increased energy requirements and changes in body composition with resistance training in older adults.

Am J Clin Nutr. 60:167–175.

8. **Pilates method**

For a good reference on the Pilates method see the website of the UK Pilates Foundation: *pilatesfoundation.com/.*

9. **Calorie-activity charts**

There are many such charts. This particular chart was based on the work of Lois Sheldahl, Ph.D, Associate Professor of Medicine at the Medical College of Wisconsin and Director of the Cardiopulmonary Rehabilitation Unit at the Milwaukee VA Medical Center, and can be found at this web link: *healthlink.mcw.edu/article/908757695.html.*

10. **American Heart Association: Benefits of exercise**

See: Statement on Exercise: Benefits and Recommendations for Physical Activity Programs for All Americans.

Circulation, 1996; 94:857–862.

Chapter 9

1. **Yom Kippur**

   For more information see: *jewfaq.org/holiday4.htm.*

2. **Catholic fasting rules during Lent**

   For more information see:
   americancatholic.org/Features/Lent/faqle9902.asp.

3. **Buddhism**

   For more information see: *buddhanet.net/e-learning/basic-guide.htm.*

4,5. **Ramadan**

   For more information see:
   bangladesh.cc/islam/new/wmview.php?ArtID=1.

6. **Fast of David**

   For more information see:
   alazhr.org/islamicpillars/Chapter4-6.htm.

7. **Fasting in Hinduism**

   For more information see:
   hinduism.about.com/library/weekly/aa041600a.htm.

8. **Ayurveda**

   For more information see: *ayur.com/about.html.*

9. **Fasting in the Mormon religion**

   For more information see
   lightplanet.com/mormons/daily/prayer/fasting_eom.htm.

Chapter 10

1. **Clive McCay**
   McCay CM, Crowell MF, Maynard LA.
   The effect of retarded growth upon the length of life span and
   upon the ultimate body size. 1935.
   Nutrition. 1989 May–Jun; 5(3):155–71; discussion 172.

2. **Mortality rate and war**
   Strom A and Jensen RA (1951) *Lancet* I, 126, 129, as cited by
   Fontana L, et al.
   Proc Natl Acad Sci USA 2004; 101:6659–6663.

3. **Okinawan centenarians and caloric restriction**
   Kagawa Y. Impact of westernization on the nutrition of Japanese:
   changes in physique, cancer, longevity and centenarians.
   Prev Med 1978;7:205–17.

4. **Dr. Walford—caloric restriction in lower animals**
   Walford RL. The clinical promise of diet restriction.
   Geriatrics. 1990 Apr;45(4):81–3, 86–7.

5. **Susan Roberts citation**
   From CNN interview. November 7, 2003. See:
   cnn.com/2003/HEALTH/11/07/calories.aging.

6. **Dr. Walford—Biosphere results**
   Walford RL, Mock D, Verdery R, MacCallum T. Calorie restriction in Biosphere 2: alterations in physiologic, hematologic, hor-
   monal, and biochemical parameters in humans restricted for a
   2-year period.
   J Gerontol A Biol Sci Med Sci. 2002 Jun;57(6):B211–24.

7. Dr. Walford citations

For more information, see: *walford.com/bio.htm*

8. Mattson data in *PNAS*

Anson RM, Guo Z, de Cabo R, Iyun T, Rios M, Hagepanos A, Ingram DK, Lane MA, Mattson MP. Intermittent fasting dissociates beneficial effects of dietary restriction on glucose metabolism and neuronal resistance to injury from caloric intake.
Proc Natl Acad Sci U S A. 2003 May 13;100(10):6216–20.

9. Caloric restriction and free radicals

See: Mattson MP, Wan R. Beneficial effects of intermittent fasting and caloric restriction on the cardiovascular and cerebrovascular systems.
J Nutr Biochem. 2005 Mar;16(3):129–37.

10. Mattson: Stress and caloric restriction

For more information, see:
usatoday.com/news/health/2003-04-28-fasting_x.htm.

11. Alzheimer and Parkinson's and caloric restriction

For more information, see:
grc.nia.nih.gov/branches/lns/mmattson.htm.

12. Perls: Book citation.

Living to 100: Lessons in Living to Your Maximum Potential at Any Age (Paperback) by Thomas T. Perls, Margery Hutter Silver, John F. Lauerman. Basic Books (January, 2000) ISBN: 0465041434.

Chapter 12

1. **Regain of weight after a diet**

   See: Anderson JW, Konz EC, Frederich RC, and Wood CL. Long-term weight-loss maintenance: a meta-analysis of US studies. *Am J Clin Nutr.,* Vol. 74(5):579–584, 2001.

APPENDIX B

QOD SNACKS AND MINI-MEALS

Veggie Juice, OJ, and Drinkable Yogurt (4 oz portions – 120 mL)

Food	Calories	cal/mL	Sodium (mg)	Potassium (mg)
Vegetable juices				
V-8™ regular, lemon, or spicy	~25	.20	300	240
V-8™ bone health	~25	.20	230	340
President's Choice 8-vegetable	~25	.20	320	240
Tomato juice	~25	.20	440	240
Orange juice and drinkable yogurt				
Orange juice	~50	.40	0	240
Non-fat Kefir (plain)	~40	.33	60	240
Low-fat Kefir (plain)	~55	.46	60	240

All values for calories, sodium, and potassium are approximate and have been rounded off to make things a bit more clear. You should take four to six 4-oz portions of tomato-vegetable juice (25 cal each) on the OFF days. The "bone health" V-8™ is nice because it has added calcium and some added potassium. It has a bit less sodium than the other V-8™ juices. The "bone health" V-8™ juice also has a more pleasing taste to some people, but this, of course, is a matter of personal preference. If you're getting tired of the taste of V-8™, try some other brands for variety. You might like the taste of the President's Choice™ vegetable juice. Diluting tomato or veggie juice with water (one part water to 3–4 parts juice) may improve the taste for people who find it too concentrated or salty. You also should take at least 4 oz of orange juice on each OFF day. Kefir/Kwashenka, from Lifeway Foods, is a drinkable yogurt. This can be consumed by itself, flavored with some cinnamon and Splenda™, or it can be used as a dressing for fruits, salads, or cold or hot vegetables. For dressings, use 2-oz portions (20-30 calories, for non-fat and low-fat, respectively). Pictures of some of the available products are reproduced below with permission. None of the companies making these products has endorsed the QOD diet, and reproduction of pictures of their products is for information purposes only.

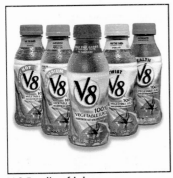

V-8 Family of juices

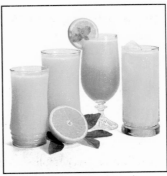

Orange juice – many brands available

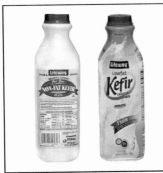

Lifeway's Kefir
(non-fat and low-fat)

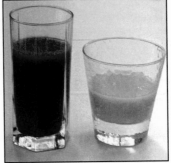

Here is a picture of an 8-oz serving of vegetable juice, and a 4-oz serving of orange juice.

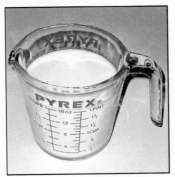

Measuring cups: Use these to learn what 4 oz and 8 oz portions of juice or yogurt look like when poured into your favorite cups and glasses.

Fruit snacks (25 cal servings)

Fruits	Calories	Grams	cal/g
Apple	25	48	0.52
Pear	25	43	0.58
Orange	25	51	0.49
Banana	25	28	0.89
Plum	25	54	0.46
Strawberry	25	78	0.32
Blueberry	25	44	0.57
Raspberry	25	46	0.52

As you can see, most fruits, except for bananas, contain about ½ calorie per gram. Because the sizes of fruits differ so much, you really need to weigh these out. Below, we picture some common fruits, weighed out to a portion size that is approximately 25–50 calories (without added yogurt dressing).

To make the dressing, use non-fat or low-fat drinkable yogurt (Kefir, unflavored). Use about 2 oz (20 or 30 calories for non-fat or low fat, respectively). Sweeten to taste using Splenda™, and add a dash of cinnamon or unsweetened lime juice for zest.

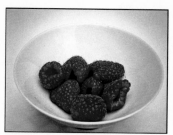

Raspberries:
24 cal, 46 g, 0.52 cal/g

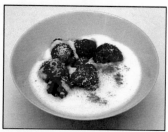

Raspberries with yogurt:
50 cal

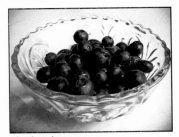

Blueberries:
40 cal, 70 g, 0.57 cal/g

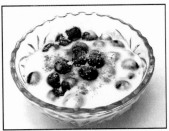

Blueberries with yogurt:
65 cal

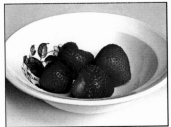

Strawberries:
25 cal, 78 g, 0.32 cal/g

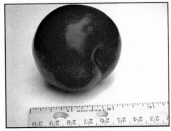

Plum:
46 cal, 92 g, 0.46 cal/g

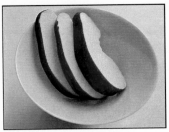

Apple slices:
25 cal, 48 g, 0.52 cal/g

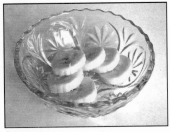

Bananas:
25 cal, 28 g, 0.89 cal/g

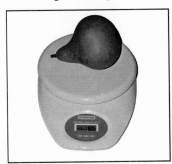

Food scale: This is one convenient food scale made by Soehnle (Myra Digital Food Scale, about $30.00). This scale has a "tare" button, so you can put a dish on the scale and zero out the scale before adding food to the dish. The food weights in this Appendix were all obtained using such a scale.

Snack vegetables (25 cal servings)

Fruits	Calories	Grams	cal/g
Pickle	25	128	0.18
Cucumber	25	167	0.15
Carrots	25	61	0.41
Radishes	25	156	0.16
Red Peppers	25	96	0.26
Green Peppers	25	125	0.20
Asparagus	25	119	0.21
Zucchini	25	156	0.16

You see here that vegetables contain only ⅓ to ½ as many calories as most fruits. Radishes and cucumbers and zucchini are best, and all of these can be eaten as crunchy snacks during the OFF day. Yogurt dressing mix: Use either non-fat Kefir (0.33 cal/mL or low-fat Kefir (0.46 cal/ml) as a dressing. Measure out about 2 oz (60 ml) of dressing (about 20-30 cal) and add salt, some lime juice, and various seasonings (dill, parsley, etc.). Other nice dressings for snack vegetables are salsa, or spaghetti sauce. Two tablespoons of salsa spread on a few Romaine lettuce leaves makes a nice 15 calorie snack (see picture below).

Here we see some pictures of approximately 15–25 cal servings of commonly available vegetables. For more info see the calorie counting websites linked via *eatQOD.com*.

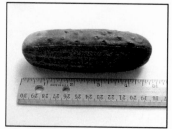

Cucumber:
17 cal, 116 g, 0.15 cal/g

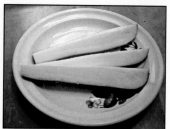

Zucchini:
25 cal, 156 g, 0.16 cal/g

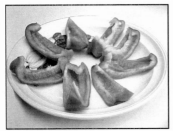

Green Peppers:
24 cal, 118 g, 0.20 cal/g

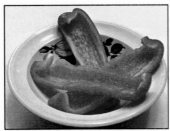

Red Peppers:
24 cal, 94 g, 0.26 cal/g

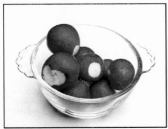

Radishes:
25 cal, 156 g, 0.16 cal/g

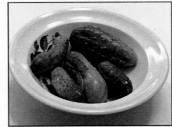

Pickles:
20 cal, 114 g, 0.18 cal/g

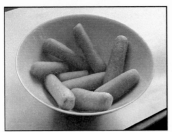

Carrots:
25 cal, 60 g, 0.41 cal/g

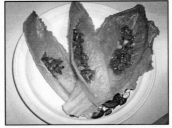

Romaine Lettuce and Salsa:
Lettuce: 6 cal, 30 g, 0.20 cal/g
Salsa: 8 cal, 30 g, (2 tablespoons)

Hot vegetable meals (20–50 cal servings)

You need to eat something in the evenings that will feel like a meal. The best strategy is to base this meal on low-calorie vegetables. The easiest way to do this is to either steam up some fresh vegetables or to get some frozen vegetables from the supermarket. Avoid frozen vegetables with sauces or with almonds. These can add a lot of calories. It is best to get vegetables without any particular type of sauce, and then make your own sauce using either drinkable yogurt or spaghetti sauce.

The quickest and easiest fresh vegetables to make are green beans, asparagus, or zucchini. The easiest vegetables to make from frozen packages are green beans, squash, zucchini, cauliflower, spinach, and mixed (yellow and green) beans. Corn, peas, lima beans, and potatoes generally have too many calories per gram to allow for a reasonable sized meal that has only 50 calories. The best way to figure out the calorie content is to look at the pack, find how many calories per serving size. Then see how many grams in the serving size. Usually vegetables will contain about 0.2–0.4 calories per gram. You can then weigh out your plate on the food scale, press the "tare" button to zero out your scale, and then add enough veggies to get about 50 calories worth. You can be creative in serving these up. I like to steam asparagus in a pan and then serve with cilantro, oregano, and a bit of lime juice. You can make "green bean spaghetti" – by using green beans just like you would pasta. Spaghetti sauce usually has few calories (check this on the label!). I also like to microwave a box of frozen squash, and then usually eat half (about 50–60 calories) flavored with nutmeg, salt, and other spices.

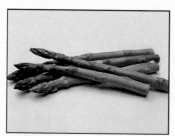

Asparagus:
20 cal, 96 g, 0.21 cal/g

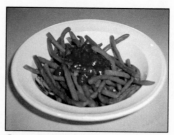

Green Beans:
40 cal, 143 g, 0.28 cal/g

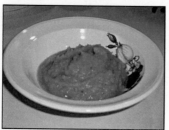

Squash:
20 cal, 125 g, 0.20 cal/g

Protein snacks (20–25 cal servings)

During your OFF day, you will be eating very little protein. You will be making up for this by eating more protein during your ON day, but it is good to eat at least 20 g of protein during your OFF day to minimize breakdown of your own body's protein. Because you will be eating very little protein, it is best to focus on "high biologic value" protein. This is protein with a good blend of amino acids. High-biologic-value protein comes from ... milk, eggs, and soybeans. If you take in 4 oz of drinkable yogurt, this will get you about 7 g. You can get another 10 g by hard boiling two eggs, and discarding the yolks. Each egg white (depending on the size of the egg) contains about 17–20 calories and 4-5 g of protein. This will bring you up to about 17 g, and the rest you will get through your vegetable juice and other foods.

"Cheater snacks" (10 calories)

During your OFF days, you will feel the need sometimes for foods from specific groups. It is OK to snack a bit, but you need to know how many calories your snacks contain, and to limit this to no more than 20-40 calories for the whole day. One potato chip, or one cracker, contains about 10 calories. A small piece of cheese sometimes hits the spot. You can weigh this out, to get 10 calories worth. A small handful of air-popped popcorn also has only 10 calories. You will need your food scale. Most nuts have about 5-6 calories per gram, so a 10-calorie cheater snack made of peanuts or walnuts will weigh only 2 g or so (that's only 2 peanuts!). Most foods like crackers or cheese or meat will have about 3-5 calories per gram – so again, only about 2-3 g portions for each snack.

Other recipes

Additional sources of recipes are linked at *eatQOD.com*.

BACK ON QOD—
A BLOGGER'S VIEW

I am including some excerpts from a blog I wrote while on a journey to lose about 22 lbs. in the course of eating QOD. This was the third time that I needed to lose weight using QOD since 1990, and each time, the weight loss was successful and the weight stayed off for many months or years.

PART One. EARLY DAYS:

Baseline weight: 209 lbs.

I'm going back on QOD. Why? For some reason, my weight has been creeping up, despite the fact that I have tried to cut out all junk food, and I have been following sort of an Atkins, mildly carb-restricted diet. I'm doing a moderate amount of walking each day, but I still spend too much time sitting or reclining while working—also 2–3 hours of TV a day (mostly watching BBC News and Charlie Rose late at night!). But still I've been taking Mookey on a daily walk. Mookey is my miniature Parti poodle. Parti stands for particouleur or "partly colored," meaning that he is part black and part white. Mookey is about 14 months old.

Apparently all of this walking and careful eating, though, is just not enough. My fighting weight has always been around 185 lbs. Lately, I've seen that creep up close to 210 lbs, and now I'm getting a jelly roll around my stomach that just has become too much.

Also, I've been having trouble concentrating on work—and I remember from the last time I went on QOD (about 2 years ago for 4 months), how eating QOD seemed to focus the mind. Nothing special today in terms of eating, but tomorrow I'm going to do it. Checked in the fridge—some vegetable juice is there, so let's do it!

My first OFF day

Day 1—Thursday, July 29th—OFF day

"A journey of a thousand deprivations begins with a single OFF day!" But in this case, I'm not particularly hungry. Had some coffee and a Fudgsicle™ with Splenda™ (100 calories), and some drinkable yogurt (8 oz, another 100 calories). Bought some Romaine lettuce—packed 9 small heads in a plastic package. Washed them all.

Around noon, started feeling a bit yucky and weak. Took the veggie juice cure—8 oz, 50 calories. Felt better right away. But needed to feel that I was crunching something. Took Romaine lettuce, spread some mayo on the inside and laid in a few pickle slices. Much better! Evening was no problem. Not a very auspicious start, but the most important thing is that I've begun.

Bread is bread, any way you slice it?

Day 2—Friday, July 30th—ON day

Ate just like normal. What I find interesting is that I'm still not really hungry for food, even after yesterday's OFF day. Tried to "listen" for specific hungers. Heated up some corn cobs in the microwave, and some frozen peas (no sauce). Then ate lots of cheese, a bowl of drinkable yogurt, which I love, two to three open-faced sandwiches. No desserts of any kind.

Interested in my bread trick? First of all, I love open-faced sand-wiches. I also like French bread-type buns. The problem is that bread itself is usually sliced way too thickly, and if you cut a bagel or a bread roll in half, you have a large piece of bread and more calories than are necessary. For this reason, when dieting, I always buy thin-sliced bread, or even better, I buy unsliced bread loaves, so I can slice off as thin a piece as I want. If I slice a French-bread style bun, some-times I get 4 slices out of it (at least 3   ad of two halves.

You ate what? This is not your father's Atkins diet!
Day 3—Saturday, July 31st—OFF day

Felt terrible this morning. Woke up with a bad headache. Since I've been drinking coffee this can't be coffee withdrawal. One thing I hadn't been doing on the treadmill at all is running—just a lot of walking. So first thing I did after doing leg stretches was to run for ½ mile at 4 miles/hr. Not fast at all. Did the trick. Felt wonderful after-ward. (The explanation may have to do with increasing the carbon dioxide level [carbon dioxide is a vasodilator] in the blood, but this is another topic).

The whole day afterward was pretty good. Started feeling a bit weak and washed out toward noon. Took some veggie juice, but also tried something different. On Romaine lettuce leaves spread some salsa dip on each Romaine lettuce leaf. Somehow the salt in the salsa and the crunchiness of the lettuce was just what the doctor ordered. OK, I have some strange tastes in food—agreed!

I know I said that the yuckies were mostly due to salt, but I still felt an uncomfortable ketotic sort of feeling plus a definite craving for some carbs. So I measured out and drank 8 oz of calcium-forti-fied orange juice (110 calories plus 27g carbs). This is not your father's Atkins diet, by any means! Also cut up and ate half of a small apple. All of this was between noon and 6 PM. After that, all hunger pangs, etc. abated and I was fine for the rest of the evening. In fact, I was marveling at how, since starting the diet, I haven't really felt HUNGRY in the true, old-fashioned sense of the word.

Mowed 1 acre of grass walking behind a powered mower—so fairly sure I've burned off more calories today than came in by far.

Dunkin' Donuts Apple Fritters—I love them!
Day 4—Sunday, August 1st—ON day

This morning got up and felt totally normal. Heated up some Stouffer's™ grilled steak and potatoes. Marvelous that this has only 220 calories! Green tea to top it off, some drinkable yogurt (8 oz) with cinnamon and a touch of maple syrup. Total calories for the big breakfast 220 plus 150 (drinkable yogurt plus maple syrup) = 400 or so, but who's counting here?

Then I did something I shouldn't. My favorite pig-out food is a Dunkin' Donuts™ apple fritter. The donut shop is only 2 miles from my home. Yes, I drove there as fast as I could. Ate the fritter and partook of their excellent coffee. Well, this time the fritter tasted *way* too sweet! So I came home disappointed, and then, after a few hours, I felt *very tired.* These large carb loads will do this to you. Curious, I looked up the caloric value of the fritter on the Dunkin' Donuts website—amazed that it was only 260 calories (glazed fritter). Anyway it's only noon and I've already put away 700 calories. But that's the program—eating a substantial amount of food in the morning. I'm not at all hungry now but a little worried about tomorrow. However, the rule is, *no anticipatory eating.* Not hungry for anything now, so I'm not eating, even though this is an ON day.

By the way, my supplements are:
–Vitamin D 800 units/day (400 may not be enough!)

–Vitamin B-12 1000 mcg/day (more than usually recommended)

–Vitamin B super complex with C

–Glucosamine (1500 mg), Chondroitin (1200 mg) Boron (3 mg) (Osteo-Biflex)

–Resveratrol (50 mg)—been reading a lot about this lately—the longevity antioxidant found in grape skins

–Cinnamon (to help metabolize glucose)

–Calcium citrate/magnesium (usually about 800 mg of calcium as supplement)

Teaspoon snacks..., Power of the sun..., Rack of ribs on the OFF day...

Day 5—Monday, August 2nd—OFF day

10:00 AM. Woke up feeling great and not at all hungry. Got out the measuring cup. No veggie juice left, so I grabbed a bottle of tomato juice. 750 mg sodium, and 450 mg (potassium) in 8 oz with only 50 calories. Measured it out and drank it. Heated up some green tea and added a dash of Vietnamese cinnamon. New idea—teaspoon snacks. *Not* heaping teaspoons, mind you. Took 1 teaspoon of (no added sodium) tomato paste (for potassium), about 5 calories. 1 teaspoon no added sugar peanut butter (just because I wanted this). 230 cal per 2 *tablespoons*, so divide by 6 (3 teaspoons = 1 tablespoon), so 40 cal there. Then 4 oz (measured this out) calcium-fortified orange juice (for its calcium and potassium content).

So total calories for breakfast were:

Tomato juice 8 oz—50
Orange juice 4 oz—55
Tomato paste 1 tsp—5
Peanut butter 1 tsp—40
Total 150

Power of the sun:

Very sunny outside. Interesting, the powers of the sun. A recent study let people use tanning booths with or without UV light (the users didn't know if the UV part of the light was on or off). The people using the booths with the UV light wanted to use it much more than those using booths with no UV light. The UV light sort of relaxed them and made them feel good. I live in a suburban neighborhood, and if you walk outside, there's not a single person around—it's as if the neutron bomb had exploded (for you nuclear war newbies, the neutron bomb is a nuclear weapon that supposedly kills all the people but leaves property intact). Anyway, there is an epidemic of vitamin D deficiency in many countries these days—since children are all inside, playing video games or watching TV.

I don't think that these mood benefits of UV light are all mediated through vitamin D (sunlight is required to convert inactive vitamin D precursors to vitamin D in the skin, and blood levels of vitamin D depend almost entirely on how much time is spent in the sun and the strength of the sun). But vitamin D has a lot of wonderful effects, not only on bone, but also on the immune system—and of interest to a 55-year old male in particular, vitamin D acts on prostate cells to prevent them from multiplying. The rate of prostate cancer is lower in parts of the country where there is more sunlight.

So I take 800 IU (international units) of vitamin D per day (packaged in those translucent yellow little jelly beans). The recommended daily dose is only 400 IU. This is part of an interesting story. High doses of vitamin D can cause harm, mainly increasing serum calcium and potentially causing calcification in the body. The minimal dose that *may* cause harm is set by regulatory bodies, and this is now set at 2000 IU per day. But there is some evidence that taking 400 IU is not nearly enough vitamin D for most people. There is some vitamin D in milk and dairy products, but usually a glass of milk will only have 100–150 IU of vitamin D in it. Research by Dr. Vieth in Toronto, Ontario (*Am J Clin Nutr.* 2001 Feb;73(2):288–94) suggested that taking 1200 IU of vitamin D appears to be safe. So this is why I take at least 800 IU of vitamin D per day (counting intake from both supplements and food). Not much of an issue now in August, in Chicago, when the sun is out, and I'm walking Mookey every day—but for many people who stay inside, or during the wintertime, low vitamin D levels can be a big problem.

Interestingly, I was in Dubai about 3 years ago, and learned that one of the groups affected with severe vitamin D deficiency is devout Muslim women—even though the sun is blazing hot, when such a woman does go outside, almost every inch of her skin is covered by her burka (a burka is a black gown that Muslim women wear).

Food specific hungers:

3:30 PM. Got real hungry around 3 PM. Heated up a pack of frozen spinach (65 calories in the whole thing, and loaded with potassium) in the microwave, and ate a third, with salt and lime juice. So about 20 calories plus 5 for the lime juice, plus added 1 tsp of tomato paste (body wanted this). Still not great, so had half a medium apple (35 calories). So now about 25 calories from the spinach and 35 from the apple half, ⸱ ⸱⸱n breakfast, so 270 calories so far for the day. The good news is, that after some more tea, feeling fine again, and it's already almost evening.

By the way, the apple never tasted so good. First evidence since starting the diet of true, food-specific hunger coming in now. The apple tasted like heaven—probably like an apple must taste to someone who's been away at sea or locked in prison. Ditto for the top of the lime that I finished eating, scraping it from the inside with my teeth. Have not enjoyed food in such a manner for a long time. Even the spinach was spot on.

Felt like I needed some protein—boiled up 2 eggs, left the yolks, and ate the whites with some spaghetti sauce—one egg white has about 4 g of protein and only 20 calories. Egg protein has high biological value—the protein intake during the OFF day is well below the amount that a person should eat on average per day (about 50 grams, at least) so if you can sneak in some high quality protein on the OFF day, so much the better.

Rack of ribs on the OFF day:

11:00 PM. The evening was fairly easy; not at all hungry, even though my wife came back from shopping and made a rack of ribs with corn on the cob. Just asked her to save me some for tomorrow. Did have a few mild hunger pangs tonight, the first since being on the diet. So strange that it took 5 full days to get back any signs of hunger. But it's not a desperate hunger or anything like that. Looking forward to tomorrow.

Morning "yuckies" during the ON day...
Day 6—Tuesday, August 3rd—ON day

9:40 AM. Slept very well, awoke feeling fine and not at all hungry. Had 3 open faced sandwiches for breakfast (bread, mayo, pâté, tomato). Also a bowl of drinkable yogurt. Interestingly, afterwards, began feeling quite weak and washed out. Tried to figure it out. My son was heating up a bowl of chicken soup—this is loaded with salt—so I poured myself half a very small bowl, and soon felt a lot better. My theory is that the low-salt yuckies begin when you get up in the morning, and spend some time in the standing position—then you need some blood volume support.

11:00 PM. Actually, felt pretty much like a normal day today. Had a fairly normal dinner at about 3 PM (chicken, potatoes)—the potatoes tasted especially good. The chicken I could actually take or leave—the specific hunger was for the potatoes. Otherwise, snacking on some plums and peaches (following specific food hungers) and peanuts in the shell. Avoiding snack foods, sugar—no particular craving for them, except just before going to bed, I had a big glass of milk and a peanut butter and jelly sandwich (open face).

Guessing calories for watermelons and why I needed a food scale...Pants getting loose, but wife prepares braised beef and it's an OFF day!
Day 7—Wednesday, August 4th—OFF day

11:00 AM. Interesting comparison to 2 days ago, when I was feeling very weak and washed out and needed salt. This AM felt totally normal. Not at all hungry. Had a slice of watermelon (because it was out there and it felt good!) and a large cup of coffee with a little bit of milk. Looked up watermelon calories at a calorie counter website. Surprisingly large amount—I thought it was mostly water, but it also has a lot of potassium. For example, 1 wedge weighing 286 grams has 86 calories, but also has 320 mg of potassium. So potassium to calorie ratio of about 4.0. This is similar to orange juice. An entire melon has 1400 calories, so if you cut it into 10 circular slices, each slice has about 140 calories. After all of this math,

I decided that I needed a food scale. Looked up digital food scales on the web. Ordered one. A must-have for serious dieters.

12:00 PM. Ran ½ mile at 4.1 miles per hour. Surprisingly easy, except for a twinge of low back pain, plus my pants started slipping down! Need to make an additional belt hole. An early sign that the diet is working already? Remarkable, after only 1 week or so. The running (and I also do Pilates) has a remarkable effect on the stomach sticking out. A little bit of abdomen goes a long way toward improving one's appearance.

Felt I needed "something" after the run. Poured a nice glass of tomato juice—ground up some black pepper on top, and I'm in heaven! My wife is in the kitchen frying up pieces of beef in a cast iron pan—I'm not the least bit interested. Feeling better today than I have been all week.

5:00 PM. My wife prepared a beautiful supper of braised beef, green beans, carrots and vegetables, and noodles. Sat down at the table with the kids. Into my plate I put 4–5 green beans, two small pieces of carrots, and about a 1-inch square of meat, and ate heartily. I estimate this was about 150 calories.

Eating weird foods on an ON day....
Day 8—Thursday, August 5th—ON day

8:00 AM. Started like a usual ON day. Not hungry at all. Had a weird breakfast. Some leftover spinach with mayonnaise (from an OFF day 3 days ago), then 2–3 watermelon slices, and I felt fine.

6:00 PM. As the day progressed, snacking from a jar of peanut butter, and had about 5–6 tablespoons of this (probably about 500 calories). A couple of sandwiches. A piece of chicken, some fruit.

Four or five slices of watermelon. Generally, feeling fine. Like I'm not on a diet at all.

Did a tremendous amount of work today—all in front of the computer while treadmill walking. Overall, today felt like a usual day—I basically ate what I wanted.

Charity Board Meeting buffet—and it's an OFF day!
Is *Helicobacter* gnawing at your soul?
The joys of radishes and asparagus...
Day 9—Friday, August 6th—OFF day

12 Noon. Woke up feeling great! Not at all hungry. Interesting day today—need to go to a meeting at 1:30 PM (lunch will be served). But it's an OFF day! So far I've only had a glass of tomato juice with a squirt of lemon. Feeling perfect. Not at all weak.

6:00 PM. I attended the Board meeting of a charitable group I belong to, and they usually have a nice tray of snacks out. This time was no different, with lovely cucumber and ham sandwiches on croissants, herring on bread—lots of hors d'oeuvres, in other words. Also some very heavy desserts, including a Napoleon cake (all butter—probably 800 calories a slice!).

At that point, I had had only two glasses of tomato juice (50 cal each), but it was very interesting—I just was *not hungry!* None of the delicious food on the tray held any attraction for me. It was wonderful! However, I had not had any calcium supplements yet, so I did try two small servings of shish-kabob'ed cheese, spinach leaf and cherry tomato (estimated calories: 30 x 2 = 60, mostly in the cheese, so 160 calories total).

Feeling wonderful, by the way. A nice clarity of mind, lots of energy, even though I haven't really had anything in the way of carbs today. The two glasses of tomato juice had done the trick. Stomach growling a bit, but not an unhealthy gnawing like I used to get before I took the *Helicobacter* cure.

Helicobacter:

The *Helicobacter* story is an interesting one. *Helicobacter pylori* is a bacterium that infects a substantial percentage of middle-aged adults in the US. Actually, the proportion of people infected increases with age, being about 50% in people my age (in their fifties). The infection rate is considerably lower in younger people. Patients infected with *Helicobacter* have a greatly increased acid secretion in their stomach, and despite a lot of initial skepticism, *Helicobacter* infection has now been linked conclusively to stomach and especially duodenal ulcers, so much so, that testing and treating ulcer patients for *Helicobacter* is now a standard of care.

A large number of people whose stomachs are colonized with *Helicobacter* have no obvious ulcer symptoms. Some, however, have what is known as "dyspepsia", defined as dysfunctional digestion—vague pains in the stomach area, etc. Whether or not killing the *Helicobacter* bugs improves the upset st‥‥ ‥‥ns is still controversial. The nice thing is that *Helicobacter* is easy to treat. A 10-day course of 2 or 3 antibiotics given along with a drug that reduces acid secretion in the stomach does the trick in more than 90% of cases. Once treated, *Helicobacter* usually does not recur. Chronic inflammation of the stomach lining by *Helicobacter* may predispose a person to exhaustion of the stomach lining (atrophic gastritis) in later years, and has been linked to a peculiar form of gastric cancer (MALT lymphoma). Since the risks are uncertain but present, and since treatment is so easy, why not treat?

Anyway, ever since my teenage years, I had gnawing pains in the upper abdomen whenever I would miss a meal. Under stress, or when I used to smoke, these would get much worse, to the point that I would be drinking antacids, or just rushing for food to make the pain go away. In later adult life, these symptoms receded, but still, if I would miss lunch, I would be uncomfortable. At that time, about 7 years ago, testing for *Helicobacter* was complicated (endoscopy) so I spent 10 days taking these antibiotics. The result for me was remarkable: I literally felt my stomach quiet down and begin to "shrink" immediately after this course of treatment. Afterward, I *never* had the gnawing pains or the feeling that I couldn't skip a meal.

Radishes and asparagus:

So I did feel my stomach gurgling today; basically, it felt empty—but no gnawing pains or discomfort.

But I felt like I needed to eat *something*. So off to the grocery store I went, looking for low-calorie veggie treats. As you recall, on the first OFF day it was Romaine lettuce; on the second OFF day it was spinach. What did I come back with? Radishes and asparagus! Looked them both up at a calorie counter website. Radishes are great. One medium-size radish—1 calorie! I took two of them, sliced each one into thirds, salted each slice, and had 6 nice crunchy bites to savor with some tea. Asparagus—medium spears—only 3–4 calories per spear. So I've only eaten 160 calories today—I'm allowing 300 calories/day on the OFF day—(you can go about 100 calories higher, especially if you exercise at least 30 min during the OFF day)—so I'm going to take about 10 asparagus spears (40 calories), cook them in a pan sprayed with Pam™, and then eat them with a snack of a tablespoon or so of tomato paste. We'll see if that will hold me.

By the way, I was thinking of buying some Splenda™ at the grocery store (sucralose). But I held off, as I have absolutely no urge for sweets.

7:00 PM. The asparagus were delicious! Salted them, and squeezed out some lemon juice over each one. Ate more tomato paste than I had planned, since it was the bottom of the can—about ⅙ of the can, or 50 calories worth. So now I'm up at 300 calories for the day.

Took Mookey for a walk. Very peaceful. This was the first OFF day that I really felt the Zen peacefulness I had encountered while trying this diet in the past. A happy calm came over me—first time in a long time. No worries, positive energy—all of the clichés, but they were there. No discomfort at all today. A happy (if mild!) ketosis, I guess. But certainly not the yucky ketosis that I had experienced while trying Atkins. In the QOD diet, you take in about 40–60 grams of carbs during the OFF day, and this is usually enough to prevent severe ketosis in most people.

Thinking about the ubiquity of food: If we eat based on habit or scheduling, then it is almost inevitable that we will overeat; there are so many social opportunities where food is involved—the family sits down to watch a movie, and the kids are passing around popcorn; a farewell party for an employee; we've eaten dinner, but guests arrive, and we have to prepare them something to eat and then we have to sit down and eat with them. You can just say no some of the time, but eating opportunities are so frequent, that even if you say no half of the time, the extra food comes in.

205 lbs. on the scale. My goal is 195. Four lbs in one week is a lot—Most of this, I'm sure, was water.

Did I already talk to you about fritters? Sugar, AGEs (advanced glycosylation end products) and sucralose…Pigging out during an ON day (dangers of bulimia and other ea⋯⋯⋯ ⋯rs)…

Day 10—Saturday, August 7th—ON day

Woke up thinking of fritters again. So this morning I went to Dunkin' Donuts,™ had coffee, read the *New York Times*, ate my fritter, and now I'm back. Now I'm not feeling so good. Not like yesterday, when Zen clarity ruled. An uncomfortable, sugar taste—a general feeling of excess. But I'm still glad I ate that fritter. Why? Because I can!

Sugar, AGEs (advanced glycosylation end-products) and sucralose:

Actually, medical evidence is accumulating that, especially in diabetics, sugary baked goods may not be good for you. Why? When you heat up a pastry with sugar, a chemical reaction takes place, creating what are called AGE, or advanced glycosylation end products. When you eat these, some of them are absorbed undigested. The bad thing about AGEs is that they can cross-link a number of molecules in the body, including collagen, making them stiffer. AGE levels in the blood, especially in diabetics, have been linked to dietary intake of AGEs. Splenda™ (sucralose), a sweetener that maintains its sweetness with cooking, may change all that, but sucralose is a chlorinated, non-metabolized derivative of sugar. What sucralose-cooked pastries contain in terms of AGEs has not been studied, to my knowledge. What eating sucralose for years will do to you is also unknown. But what the naturopaths and chiropractors have been saying about sugar being bad for you may be partially true, and one of the connecting links may be the AGEs that are present in sugary baked pastries, and also the AGEs that a high-sugar diet can create simply by increasing the glucose level in the blood. Is all of this enough to keep me from eating fritters? Not really—especially if the local Dunkin' Donuts™ wises up and starts offering the kind that contains a delicious apple compote center.

By the way, eating such "junk" food on the ON day makes it tough to get enough potassium. Potassium is a wonder mineral. Higher dietary intakes of potassium have been linked to lower blood pressure, a healthier cardiovascular system, a lower rate of stroke, and even, when potassium is combined with an alkali, with better bone density. The suggested daily requirement is 4–5 g/day, and there is no way that you can get there during your OFF day with 2–3 glasses of tomato and orange juice. You need to eat a lot of potassium-rich fruits and vegetables on the OFF day, and you also have to make sure that you take in lots of potassium on your ON day, by eating enough dairy and fruits and vegetables. Again, calcium-fortified orange juice is a great way to get a lot of both potassium and calcium.

One thing that should be avoided for anyone going on a diet (and probably for people in general), is glucose-sweetened soft drinks. Even those sweetened with artificial sweetners are probably not that good for people. The soft drinks sweetened with sugar are bad because they give an unnaturally quick load of refined sugar to the body, which causes a spike in insulin; plus a high sugar intake contributes to increasing the amount of AGEs in the body; plus you have carb craving. Not only that, soft drinks are very expensive. Fast food outlets, I am told, sell their burgers and meats pretty much at cost, and they make much of their money from the profits on selling soft drinks and fries, which are cheap to produce. Our own family just asks for water at these restaurants, and the bill (there are 6 of us) is cheaper by 6–10 dollars as a result

Pigging out during an ON day (dangers of binge eating and other eating disorders):

11 PM. This is not a day I was proud of. First of all, I spent pretty much the whole day on the couch, watching TV with the kids or surfing the web. Only exercise I got was my usual walk with Mookey— thank God for the dog! Corn chips with avocado dip, and on and on, until the evening, capped off with a nice serving of fresh-baked

banana bread. Lot's of semi-useless activity, and I didn't get much useful work done, although it was a nice and relaxing day—probably a
typical American Saturday, unfortunately. This is the reason we
Americans, and in fact the entire developed world, are becoming
obese. Television, and now the internet, and a cornucopia of delicious
food just steps away. In my defense, I did stay away from soft drinks
and ice cream, which my boys were happily downing in addition to
the stir fry (oh and I forgot about the s...   ...-year-old and
14-year-old made, with chicken, orange slices, rice, and Thai peanut
sauce that was done to perfection!). Of course I tried some!

Today, I must have eaten more than 3000 calories, and that
would be terrible, were it not for the fact that, at 6'4" tall, my
expected energy intake when not dieting is about 2500–2800 calories per day. But it was a bit too much food, even for an ON day. Most
importantly, I was violating a cardinal rule of the diet—instead of
eating because I was hungry, and eating only those foods that I was
hungry for, I was eating just for the sake of eating—out of conven-
ience, socializing, and just because the food was there.

A number of unfortunate people suffer from a syndrome called
bulimia, where they eat and eat and eat without rhyme or reason, and
sometimes to great excess. This is highly dangerous, and there are
reports of people suffering a sudden heart attack after eating a large,
calorie- and fat-rich meal. Also, sometimes such people get the idea
that they can eat a lot and then stick a finger in their throat and throw
up all of their food—sort of eating their cake and not having it! Again,
this is a highly dangerous, addictive sort of behavior. The repeated
vomiting sometimes causes people to completely goof up the control
between acids and bases in the blood, and also these people sometimes get depleted potassium. If you have any tendency to these sorts
of eating disorders, then the QOD diet plan is definitely NOT for you.

The opposite problem: restricting foot too much on the ON day:

There's a reverse problem that can occur during QOD eating.
You can find that partial fasting is so easy that it may be tempting to
also not eat too much on the ON day. I think it's a mistake to restrict

food too much on the ON day, since the body may interpret this as a famine situation and start to downregulate the metabolic rate.

You put the lime in the coconut and mix it all up... or on your berries that you eat with yogurt. Dinner at mother's during an OFF day...

Day 11—Sunday, August 8th—OFF day

Woke up this morning feeling fine. Went to Church from 9–10 not having eaten anything. Absolutely no problems. As a kid, I remember that we would always go to Church on Sunday on an empty stomach, since it was thought that to receive Holy Communion on a full stomach was not a proper way of receiving that Sacrament. Then all of the rules liberalized and changed. However, I've noticed that Sunday Mass is much better on an empty stomach. Somehow it was easier to compose myself and follow the service on an empty stomach.

Teaching my son to drive, so we stopped off at our local grocery store for ingredients—meal planning for my 300-calorie OFF day. Bought some more lettuce and radishes. Also bought fresh raspberries and blueberries, plus some Splenda™ (sucralose) in granular form, plus some lime juice (no sugar added, no calories).

To vary the pace, I thought it would be nice to make a nice 40-calorie snack. Looked up raspberries and blueberries on a calorie counter website. Basically, 20 calories per 100 g. By now I had received the food scale that I had ordered. I used it to weigh the contents of the pack of raspberries I had bought—the berries in the plastic tray weighed 170 grams; I put half of them into in a bowl (so about 15 calories worth of raspberries), and put in 50 mL (¼ cup) of drinkable yogurt, which has about ½ calorie per ml, so about 25 calories. 25 + 15 = 40. Added cinnamon (which helps insulin act to metabolize sugars), and sprinkled about a teaspoon of granular Splenda™ on top. Tasted wonderful, and it was a nice respite from the veggies.

Dinner at mother's:

11:00 PM—Got invited up to my mother's house for dinner. Had a mini-lunch—I was going to do something special, but did the asparagus (10 small spears, 40 cal)/tomato sauce (30 cal), radishes (2–3 cal) bit again.

Dinner was interesting. We had a marinated pork roast, potatoes, salad, green beans, cauliflower, white wine, and cognac. Some great discussions with my brother, who is a champion of the Atkins diet. What to do? I'm sitting in front of all of this wonderful food, and it's an OFF day—and I had only about 150 calories remaining to eat! Well, I ate mostly salad (with yogurt dre.... .....out 8–9 green beans, and a small piece of cauliflower. I also snacked on some of the clear meat gravy (about 2 tablespoons) which was very satisfying. So I figure that I ate only 100 calories, tops. Of course we had to drink wine and make a few toasts; A glass (3.5 fl oz) of white wine has 70 cal (checked on a calorie counter website)—I just poured myself about ⅓ of a glass and that was it for the meal. With the brandy, it was more problematic. This has 70 cal in only 1 fl oz. So I had just a taste. All in all, dinner went very well. I greatly enjoyed the spirited conversation, participated in the toasts, and restricted myself to about 200 calories—didn't miss the meat and potatoes at all (of which I ate none, of course!).

Just another ON day...

Day 12—Monday, August 9th—ON day

Woke up feeling very fine. Took calcium supplements and a piece of banana bread that was hanging around all day yesterday (when I couldn't eat it!). Typical ON day—no hunger whatsoever in the morning. Trying to get some work done before eating a big breakfast.

Spent the entire day working on the computer in a room next to the kitchen. Food was in abundance, and I basically ate what I wanted. We didn't really have a complete supper—so I was eating primarily sandwiches, including some with cheese melted on the top. Plus, my wife cooked up some red peppers in the oven, she somehow soaks these in oil, so they make an excellent sandwich topping. Also a few nectarines. I guess I should be counting calories, but I'm just relying on common sense.

Blueberries, cinnamon, apples, green beans, tomato paste, and tuna (not all at once!)

Day 13—Tuesday, August 10th—OFF day

Weighed myself today, and only weighed 203 lbs. So that's a 6 lb weight loss in about 10 days. Seems like a lot. Felt fine, as usual during the OFF days. Had some coffee with cinnamon, and then, around noon, a glass (8 oz) of veggie juice. So I came into the noon break with only 50 calories spent. Had some blueberries (fresh) so I wanted to repeat the raspberry experiment of a few days ago. Counted out 20 blueberries (15 calories), and added 60 mL of drinkable yogurt (30 calories), so now add 45 calories to the total.

4 PM. Feeling great in general. Working while walking on the treadmill and talking on the phone—doing a lot of computer design work for my website. About an hour ago, took a medium apple, cut it in two and then in two again. This quarter-of-an-apple contains about 17 calories. I sliced it into 3 pieces, and drizzled some cinnamon on each slice. Had this with some coffee with a touch of milk. As delicious as apple pie!

6 PM. Now feeling a bit weak. Took another 8 oz of veggie juice, and then decided it was time for "supper." This time, I opened up a pack of frozen green beans with sliced almonds (no sauce). Put the almonds aside, since they are loaded with calories, unfortunately. We'll save these for an ON day. The whole 200 g pack of green beans (without the almonds) has only 70 calories. After heating took ½ of this, added 2 tablespoons of spaghetti sauce, and sprinkled it with lime juice and pepper. Tasted great. Not unlike a spaghetti dinner! So 35 calories from beans, 30 from the spaghetti sauce.

Oh, by the way, I saw a can of open tuna on the counter (tuna in oil, 150 calories in the can), and took a small smidgeon (less than ⅒ of the can, believe me!), so another 15 calories there. Plus, I admit, there was a very small boiled potato on the counter—took about a teaspoon size piece with my veggie juice (these potatoes, unfortunately, are loaded with calories). A good lesson—it's better to just stay out of the kitchen on the OFF days.

Eating peach pie late in the evening and thinking about weight loss...

Day 14—Wednesday, August 11th—ON day

Woke up feeling fine, as usual, not particularly hungry. Heated up a Stouffer's Healthy Meal™—beef goulash (320 cal). Cut 3 slices of black bread, and spread mayo and added a slice of cheese. So I've only been up and about for an hour or so, and already I've put away several hundred calories. But this is fine 3. according to plan. During the ON day, you want to eat like farmers do: Full breakfast, a relatively large lunch, and then a smaller supper. Again, *No anticipatory eating!* Eat only when you're hungry, and what you're hungry for. This works much better if you surround yourself with a variety of foods from different food groups, so that you can sort of look at the refrigerator and identify whatever particular food your body is craving. It is *impossible* to do this if all you have around is junk food. And, of course, even on the ON day, no sugared soft drinks, and a limit of one pastry item for the entire day.

Around bedtime, though, my son and I cooked up a deep-dish peach pie. This has an amazing number of calories—about 3400 for the whole pie. Had two ⅙ slices, so about 800 calories at 10 PM. Not what I recommend: eating a lot in the late evening is not good for you, since eating stimulates secretion of stomach acids, and when you lie in bed flat, especially if you're a back sleeper, the acids wash back into your esophagus, and you can get a fairly bad case of heartburn leading to esophagitis. But that was 10 PM, and it's 1 AM now.

By the way, I weighed myself a few hours ago—206 lbs. And it was 203 a day or two ago. So it's important to know that, whenever you weigh yourself, it's going to be plus or minus about 3 pounds, depending on how full your stomach is, when you last emptied your bowels and bladder, and so on. This actually is more in line with the 1–2 lb weight loss that one should expect with most diets. You need to be patient. I remember the last time I was on QOD, the weight loss also seemed to drop in steps. You need to take an average.

Peach pie last night, heartburn this morning… The joys of squash, green tea, and lime juice…

Day 15—Thursday, August 12th—OFF day

11 AM. Woke up with a tiny bit of heartburn this morning. This is what happens when you break the rules (the rule is: don't eat a fairly large meal after 7 PM, or within 4 hours of going to sleep). Was the peach pie worth it? Don't know. Still have a sugary aftertaste from it (obviously imagination). Looking forward to a clear, relaxing day today, and getting a lot of work done. Only a cup of coffee so far. Yesterday I was eyeing a package of frozen squash—in fact had a "specific hunger" for it, but was too lazy to prepare it. Today that frozen squash (at least half of it) is mine!

6 PM. Very busy all day—too busy to eat, so I relied on the old standby—veggie juice. A glass around 11 AM and another around 4 PM and that's it for 100 calories. Heated up a package of squash— 135 calories. Spiced it up with some nutmeg, a touch of curry, and cut up 3–4 scallion tubes for flavor. Ate the whole thing, assuaging a specific hunger for squash that I first experienced the night before. So now I'm up to 235 calories. Wish I had some berries—because I feel like the raspberry/blueberry drinkable yogurt 50-calorie snack now would really hit the spot—but the berries are no more.

So I settled for 100 mL (measured out) of drinkable yogurt (50 calories) with cinnamon and Splenda.™ Still needed something to crunch on, so I grabbed a stick of celery. Much later, had some green tea flavored with a hint of with lime juice and cinnamon and sweetened with Splenda.™ Finally I'm done -eating- with 25 calories to spare.

Well, not quite done—about 9 PM I ate two potato chips (10 calories per chip)! And that about did it.

Has my stomach been shrinking? It's an ON day and I can't finish up my American-portion size meal at the restaurant…

Day 16—Friday, August 13th—ON day

11 PM. Nothing unusual to report today. Woke up late, ate a sandwich with roast beef. About 1 PM took the kids to a neo-Greek restaurant. Ordered a ½ lb burger—hungry for meat. But when I got

it, I was surprised that I wanted the coleslaw more than the meat. Ate most of the burger, anyway, but I was surprised that I could barely eat the whole thing. This would not have been a problem 3 weeks ago. I believe that the stomach "shrinks" somewhat during the OFF days, so that these huge American-style meals get less comfortable to eat. The whole family had only water to drink at the restaurant, by the way.

Later in the day, just had a salad. Not really hungry. Then my wife baked some oatmeal cookies—had about ~~~~~~ ~~~~~ ~~ese, I'm sorry to say—sort of violates the carb-craving rule. Also snacked on some cheese corn while watching the opening ceremonies of the Olympic Games in Athens. No treadmill today. One downside of the diet is that you do feel a bit more lethargic and tired on the ON days. It must be a bit of work for the body to digest food! But as I was explaining to my son, the nice thing about QOD is that the OFF days are doable, and on the ON days, you just eat like a regular person. Anyway, it was interesting that I seemed to be needing carbs today, much more so than meat or vegetables. But this is *not* the Atkins diet—so why not have a few carbs?

Coffee and chocolate: good or bad?
Day 17—Saturday, August 14th—OFF day

3 PM. Feeling OK, but not great. Part of the not feeling great is that I missed coffee this AM. Need to go out and get some bottled water. After some more caffeine, everything should be fine. Brewed myself two large cups, and after an hour or so, the sleepiness and "not there" feeling went away. Coffee is a powerful stimulant. If you have even 1 cup after having stopped taking in coffee for a week or so, coffee will cause a marked increase in heart rate and increase in blood pressure, and the stimulant effect will be very strong. Drink coffee every day for 1 week or so, and then your body gets used to the coffee, and after drinking a cup or two, changes in heart rate and blood pressure are much less pronounced. But for me, anyway, if I suddenly stop drinking coffee, I often get headaches and feel very slow and drowsy. In fact, I think that's why headache pill manufacturers like the caffeine in their headache pills. Stop taking the pill

and the headache comes back! So one of the rules of QOD-ing is, if you are a coffee drinker, don't stop drinking coffee on your OFF day. You should stop using sugar if you like your coffee sweet, and switch to Splenda.™ Also, you can use milk, but only up to one tablespoon, since this already contains about 7–10 calories. One caveat: Coffee can make you lose salt and water because it acts like a diuretic, so no more than 1–2 cups/day.

Chocolate: Good or bad?

I am still not sure about chocolate. Chocolate is basically healthy for you and has anti-oxidants and may actually help prevent heart disease! Scientists have shown that chocolate makes you feel good partly by stimulating opiate receptors, the same receptors that are stimulated by morphine and opium! On the other hand, chocolate has lots of oxalate in it—to the point that, if you take a large amount before going to bed, and if you are a little bit dehydrated, the oxalate level in your urine might get too high and you might get a kidney stone. Or maybe only kidney doctors worry about such things! Nothing like a large mug of hot water, cocoa (unsweetened cocoa powder only!) and added Splenda™ to make it sweet! I can't make up my mind. I love this chocolate so!

Sleepy with spaghetti—it's all the pasta's fault!
Day 18—Sunday, August 15th—ON day

9 AM. 201.5 lbs. Woke up feeling rather weak and not very good. On weighing myself was very surprised: 201 lbs only! I think this was why I was feeling poorly last night and especially this morning. When you don't eat and get ketotic, you excrete ketones in your urine, and this acts like a diuretic—(a diuretic is anything that enhances excretion of urine). Coffee is also a diuretic, and the two probably worked together to cause the difference in weight today vs. yesterday.

Had a glass of tomato juice and coffee plus two large glasses of water and felt fine.

11 PM. Had a good day today. Ate two open-face roast beef sandwiches, spaghetti that my wife prepared around 11 AM for everyone,

a couple of low calorie ice-cream pops, drinkable yogurt, orange juice. And a hot dog around 9 PM. How many calories? Wasn't counting, but probably still under 3000. Felt very sleepy after the spaghetti. Lots of carbs today. Actually, I had a specific hunger for some fruit, especially an apple, but we didn't have any in the house.

Just weighed myself again: 205.5 lbs. Not happy with this 4 lb difference in weight in the course of one day. Of course some of this was due to the spaghetti—but I think ~~he~~ ~~~~ ~~~~n was too much salt and water loss yesterday—and maybe too little salt and water intake. I intend to follow this more closely tomorrow.

Anyway, this shows how hard it is to follow your weights while on a diet. Usually you expect to lose about 1 lb per week. So after 17–18 days on QOD, I'm quite happy to be in the 205 lb range now. Remember that I started out at around 210 lbs, so this means about 1–2 lbs of weight loss per week.

Daily weight fluctuations during QOD and for the rest of us...
Day 19—Monday, August 16th—OFF day

9 AM. Got interested in the weight issue, so I weighed myself first thing on getting up. 203.5 lbs, compared with 205.5 last night. There are 4 reasons for weight loss overnight: First, you burn glycogen, and this contains a lot of water, which you exhale in your breath. Second, you have additional "insensible" water loss in your breath that continues while you are sleeping and is not counteracted by way of drinking. Third, when you sleep, you raise your legs, so blood flows back to your kidneys, so that they may make a bit more urine. Fourth, if you are fasting for a long enough time and severely enough to develop slight ketosis, this tends to make your kidneys excrete more salt and water.

Pants are getting looser...
Day 20—Tuesday, August 17th—ON day

Ate a lot today: Two sandwiches, a couple of hot-dogs. Had a small Dairy Queen™ soft cone with my son. Cooked up a hamburger for dinner. Seemed to have a craving for orange juice—again, certainly not low-carb. Also ate an ice cream bar—why not? No exercise—had to drive my son to several different places—no time on the treadmill or even to walk the dog. Feeling good. Again, this is a lot of food, but really I've eaten as much when not dieting. Ran out of tomato juice. Will have to get some to help get through tomorrow.

Pants are getting looser, and the flab around my stomach is noticeably smaller. Will keep trying to weigh myself in the morning and evening and graph it. Looking forward to getting below 200 lbs.

PART TWO: Extracts

OK, I'm sure that you're getting bored reading this daily blog. I did keep it every day for the first 2 months that I was on QOD. Here are some highlights of my musings from some of the later entries. And here is the weight loss chart, if you don't remember it from Chapter 9.

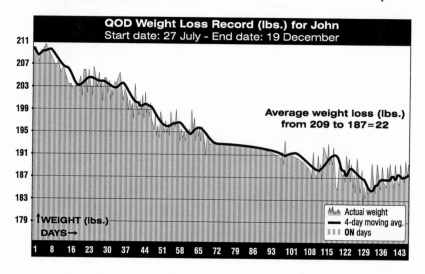

QOD saves me: Deep-fry party during an OFF day…

Day 23—Friday, August 20th—OFF day

11 PM. Went to see a movie. When we came back, a deep-frying party going on. The kids were experimenting with a new deep fryer that we had just bought—deep frying Hostess Twinkies—some sort

of cult food—as well as pieces of chicken. I'm *so* glad this was my OFF day—otherwise, I would have put away 1500 calories or more for sure. Hey—this is another benefit of QOD—you have a 50% chance that a potential pig-out feast happens on an OFF day, an additional form of protection! I still had about 150 calories left. Spent it by measuring out 100 mL of orange juice and 100 mL of drinkable yogurt. Then I nibbled on some lettuce, some tomatoes, and before retiring, a small plum (about 20 calories). I ac̲ ̲   ̲ ̲ine, eating my drinkable yogurt, OJ, and some salad.

Taking some salty foods during the morning of the ON day...
Day 24—Saturday, August 21st—ON day

9 AM. Weighed 201 this morning. Felt fine, but I decided that I needed some salt. When on QOD, theoretically, a person will be the most salt-depleted on the morning of the ON day. Why? Because during the OFF day, despite tomato juice, sodium intake will be only about 2 g/day. Also, there may be some ketosis, which tends to make you lose salt. This is reflected by the weight chart, which shows the lowest weights the morning of the ON day.

It is important to recognize this and not to start eating everything in sight because of a vague feeling of the blahs on the ON day. Also, eating will cause the blood vessels around the intestines to dilate, and some of the blood in the circulation is used to fill these expanded vessels. So if you eat something the morning of the ON day that has no salt; you might feel even worse. The correct move is to take something a bit salty the morning of the ON day. Tomato juice would be fine, but you can get tired of drinking this every day. So this morning I had a small piece of fried chicken and some potato chips. Also a half-glass of orange juice, and I feel great.

You don't want to take too much salt on the ON day, though. Normally, as I've said before, Americans eat way too much salt, 3000–4000 mg of sodium per day. It is somewhat controversial whether or not this is bad. But it is clear that this much salt is bad for some people, including the elderly, most people with high blood pressure, people with kidney disease, and many African

Americans and Hispanics, whose ancestors were never exposed to a higher salt diet.

You certainly should not get into the habit of saying: I feel bad— need some more salt! Feeling badly, having the yuckies, etc. can have many causes. And you should be keeping track of the sodium you are taking in. Even if you are perfectly healthy, eating way too much sodium may be bad for you.

11:30 PM. Weight: 205 lbs.

Getting tired of the taste of veggie juice...
Being sociable at dinner during an OFF day...
Day 27—Tuesday, August 24th—OFF day

Woke up feeling fine. Just coffee and one glass of veggie juice around 11 AM. About ½ hr. ago, started to feel a bit so/so. Took a second glass of spicy veggie juice. Again, getting tired of the taste. Need to find some alternative high-sodium, high-potassium vegetable drink. For the moment, since I love tomatoes, regular tomato juice is still fine.

5 PM. For dinner my wife made cod filets with green beans, and tomato salad, plus spaghetti. I had 200 calories to go, so to be sociable, took ⅓ piece of cod without the hollandaise sauce (2 oz, about 25 calories), about 4 oz of salad (mostly cherry tomatoes with some greens for flavor), with a yogurt sauce (25 calories), and then about 4–5 pieces of cut green beans. So a total of 60 calories. Made little hors d'oeuvres, starting from a pickle slice, about ½ teaspoon of cod or a quarter section of cherry tomato. The pickles were used to increase the salt content, since the fish was otherwise not salted. Then for dessert measured out 200 mL of drinkable yogurt with cinnamon and Splenda™ (80 calories). So up to 240 calories for the day, now. Feeling fine.

Feeling thinner...
Can Zen conquer raspberry pancakes?
Day 29—Thursday, August 26th—OFF day

9 AM. Weight: 200.5 lbs.

The good news is I definitely feel thinner. Interesting how this weight loss appears to come in steps. I feel as if I had taken off an overcoat—a different, thinner person—one who needs less food, and who is more "together." Hard to describe, but a good feeling.

Can Zen conquer raspberry pancakes?

7 PM. Got a bit hungry around five-ish—had another 8 oz of veggie juice (with added lemon-lime) and 4 oz drinkable yogurt with cinnamon and Splenda™ (with 4 added fresh raspberries!). Felt absolutely wonderful. During daily walk with   back into the Zen thing again with deep thoughts. Interestingly, my wife was making gourmet pancakes with raspberries, but the food had absolutely no draw or power over me. One of the nice things about QOD is that it allows one to reset his or her relationship with food; certainly on the OFF day the relationship is dispassionate—so nice to have an evening where you don't have to take an hour off to prepare, eat and cleanup a large supper, and then to feel bloated and tired afterward. Snacked on a single raspberry after we got back from the walk, savored the taste of this single berry greatly, without wanting more.

My feeling overall is one of impatience. I feel that I have shed one "skin" of abdominal fat—I want to hurry up and shed the rest.

Wedding etiquette when it's an OFF day; not eating everything on your plate.

Day 31—Saturday, August 28th—OFF day

9 AM Weight: 203.0 lbs.

Interesting day. Invited to a wedding at 6 PM. So I just had two 8 oz glasses of veggie juice (50 cal each), one in the morning, and one around 2 PM. So I was going into the wedding with 200–300 calories left. Careful to take vitamins and calcium supplements, but no drinkable yogurt, orange juice, or veggies today, to leave some options open for the wedding meal.

Meanwhile, I felt great right up until it was time to leave for the wedding. In fact, I was very busy all day and forgot about food, and had that nice Zen-fast feeling all day.

Reception started at 6:00 PM. Asked the bartender for soda water, and then diet Coke.™ A champagne toast of course, but just several sips; same for red wine. For the meal, ate half a cup of the soup (40 cal), half of the salad with dressing (probably around 60 cal), and a small taste only of the huge piece of rice-stuffed chicken. I did eat several tablespoons of the vegetables, which were mostly red and green peppers, with eggplant, stir fried in oil. Here it's tough to calculate, but I'm sure that I ate enough to make up the final 200 calories allowed. A few strawberries thrown in for dessert.

A bit awkward, to leave the huge piece of chicken and potato on the plate largely untouched, but a number of people, especially the women, were apparently also unable or unwilling to eat such a large chunk of meat. You need to get used to leaving food on your plate, particularly if you're not really hungry for it. Too many of us were trained as children to "finish everything on your plate!"

Breaking the fat barrier: Below 200 lbs for the first time in a long time—but this lasted for about 12 hours!

Day 32—Sunday, August 29th—ON day

9 AM Weight: 199.5 (woo hoo! :-)

Woke up feeling fine. A bit tired. Celebrating the first breaking of the 200-lb barrier in a long time. I realize that it will be at least 3–4 more weeks until the *evening* weight on the ON day falls below 200—still, during the past month, my weight was never below 200.

Otherwise, interesting breakfast. Had a sandwich (open faced, bread, deli meat, cheese, tomatoes, radishes, mayonnaise) and then felt unsatisfied—craving a glass of veggie juice. Took this and felt better, then craving a tablespoon of flax seeds. The specific hungers mode is kicking in. I am becoming reacquainted with eating what the body needs.

By the way, another party scheduled for tonight—my mother's birthday. So QOD does prevent back-to-back overeating at such functions.

All morning, I've been craving, surprisingly, green beans and spinach. Unfortunately none in the house. Substituted with broccoli and peppers from some stir fry in the frig. The party began at 6 PM—

my wife is a wonderful cook, so I ate with gusto including two pieces of cake, wine, cognac—what a life!

11 PM weight: 205 lbs (oops!) But being below 200 was great while it lasted!

In praise of duck and mayonnaise...
Day 36—Thursday, September 2nd—ON day

7 AM. Weight: 198.5 lbs (woo hoo!)

Ok, I skipped writing about yesterday's OFF day—because it was not very interesting. Today was another ON day. Started out with half-glass of tomato juice and a banana (bought yesterday). Had some leftover duck from 2 days ago, a piece of back and a piece of leg, dipping each piece into about 2 tbsp of mayonnaise. OK—this is not the typical breakfast, but it does fall into the principles of QOD—eat mostly of what you are specifically hungry for. Mayonnaise is one of my favorite foods—it is soy-oil based, so it is polyunsaturated, and the high fat content does wonders for satiating hunger. I use it all the time in sandwiches and almost never use butter or margarine (with the exception, of course for "sweet" sandwiches, such as bagel/butter/walnuts/honey). Duck is high fat, but from my Eastern European (Lithuanian) heritage, duck fat was prized as a health remedy—my mother-in-law even uses it on her hands to prevent dryness! Then I did have a few sandwiches. Used the bagel trick—slicing a half-bagel in half again to make two sandwiches, and always making sandwiches open-faced, to limit the amount of bread.

Now, 5 weeks into QOD, first of all, I am very happy with the changes in the amount of abdominal fat—my pot belly is a lot smaller, although it still has room to reduce. Also, my eating patterns on the ON day have been changing. At the beginning I was eating a bit more food during the ON days than usual. Now I am eating pretty much as I used to eat when I was eating every day, but the food selection is changing. I find that I am not at all attracted to junk foods, cakes, cookies (OK, I did eat one cookie this morning!).

I feel fine, but a bit tired, as I noticed while walking Mookey. I actually feel better on my OFF days than on my ON days—it seems to take energy to digest this food.

11 PM. Weight 200 lbs.

Under 200 for sure, and I really mean it...
Day 37—Friday, September 3rd—OFF day

9 AM. Weight: 198.5 lbs.

11 PM. Weight: 199.5—this is the first *evening* weight below 200! After 37 days, I really feel a sense of accomplishment. For the first time, I am able to control my weight and not the other way around. However, I realize that I am *still* 15 pounds heavier than the weight that I always used to keep. But it's definitely a moment to mark and celebrate!

The joys of a smaller-capacity stomach...
Day 38—Saturday, September 4th—ON day

9 AM. Weight: 197 lbs.

Had a small sandwich, then went to a friend's funeral Mass and wake. Buffet lunch at the wake—not feeling very hungry, but ate reasonably well. Then dinner at my mother's which is always copious and delicious. Had three (small) pieces of fruit tart, and my stomach was bursting at the seams. Not that I ate more than I usually do at these dinners, but I noticed, since starting QOD, that my stomach must have shrunk, because I physically can't stuff in the same amount of food that I used to.

Fat cells a-poppin'? Must be my imagination...
Day 40—Monday, September 6th—ON day

9 AM. Weight; 197.5 lbs.

Not feeling particularly hungry. Had a sensation of my abdominal fat melting away in bed last night. A prickly feeling around abdomen (ok—call me crazy—I feel those fat cells a-poppin'!). I don't want to get too much into this before I destroy my credibility, but I do feel some very subtle prickles around my abdominal area, almost always the night after the OFF day. Liposuction the old fashioned way?

Weight loss picking up speed...
Day 46—Sunday, September 12th—ON day

7 AM. Weight: 195 lbs.

I'm surprised by the fact that my weight seems to be dropping more quickly now. In retrospect, the Olym   ys were spent mostly on the couch watching the show, were probably partly to blame. I'm also eating less on my ON days, mostly because I'm just not that hungry, and specific food hungers are kicking in.

Weak during an ON day morning—saved by a little brat...
Day 49—Tuesday, September 14th—ON day

9 AM weight: 193.5

Felt terrible this morning—weak, washed out. So to repeat, the time you get salt-depleted on QOD the most is the morning of the ON day. Why? Ketosis from yesterday's OFF day, coupled with the relatively lower salt intake can lead to some salt and water depletion

So I ate half a bratwurst. This is "unhealthy" food, and usually contains about 800 mg of sodium per sausage. Then I heated up a corn on the cob and ate this with butter and salt. Finally, I had 8 oz of orange juice. The result? 30 minutes later, I felt fine.

8 PM. Weight: 198 lbs.

Plateau in the weight loss again...
Day 56—Tuesday, September 21st—OFF day

9 AM. Weight: 195.5 lbs.

Interesting how the weight seems to have plateaued, but this is how weight-loss seems to progress—none for a week or two, then a sudden drop, and then another plateau. So don't get discouraged—you really have to look at a 4-day moving average of your weight loss chart to see what's going on.

11 PM. Weight: 196 lbs.

Weight loss begins anew and another fat cells a-poppin' night..
Day 57—Wednesday, September 22nd—ON day

9 AM. Weight: 193 lbs.

Another fat cells a-poppin' night. This morning had a double baloney sandwich with cheese, and then some poppy-seed rolls—got very hungry for green vegetables—heated up a package of snow peas in the pods—I have to remember this for the OFF day—only 50 calories.

11 PM. Weight: 195 lbs.

Is something wrong? Why aren't you eating?
Day 60—Saturday, September 25th—OFF day

9 AM. Weight: 194.5 lbs

9 PM. Weight: 195 lbs.

Went to a sit-down official dinner—made the mistake of ordering tonic water thinking it had no calories—it was too sweet. Had some salad and mostly vegetables—passed on the grated potatoes and chicken and sliced pork. Passed on the various dessert table cakes—had a few strawberries, but had a great time. The only annoying thing was the person sitting next to me who, between shoveling sausage, chicken, rice, and mashed potatoes into his plate, kept asking me: "What's wrong? Why aren't you eating?"

To make a long story short...

Basically, as you can see from the chart, I continued on QOD through the fall, and even through a 5-day conference that took place in another city. I arranged my ON/OFF schedule so that I could eat well during Thanksgiving, and the Christmas holiday, and I avoided the usual holiday weight gain.

My weight kept going down until my average weight was about 185 lbs. This was a 24-lb overall weight loss from the time that I started. I did feel that this amount of weight loss was a bit too much, and I then allowed myself to climb back up into an average weight of about 188 lbs, where I feel the most comfortable. I stopped the diet in January.

Update and follow-up

It is now September of the following year, 14 months after I started the QOD diet. Between February and July, my weight did creep back up to the 194–197 range. Interestingly, this happened even after I started to go to the health club every day and swim—swimming makes you so hungry! So, to tune up, went back on QOD about 8 weeks ago. Right now my weight is at the 184–188 range, more or less just where I want it, although I may   about 4 more pounds. I'm still swimming every day now, OFF day and ON day. Eating QOD is even easier this time around, since I've come up with more food choices. I'm taking in 8 g of fiber supplement every day, and most importantly, I'm drinking at least 32 oz of water each day (especially on the OFF days). Also, I'm allowing myself 50–100 "cheater calories" on the OFF days while swimming, and this is making the OFF days quite a bit easier to live through. So I'm confident that I can easily lose the weight and stay where I want to be by applying QOD once in a while.

It's been fun and interesting, and I hope that eating QOD can work for you as well as it has for me.

FEEDBACK FORM

Please mail to:
White Swan Publishing, Ltd.
15W560 89th St.
Willowbrook, IL 60527

Or: Email to:
feedback@whiteswanbooks.com

General comments about the book or the QOD diet:

_____
_____
_____
_____

Problems or question? (If you want a response, please include con-
tact info, preferably email)

_____
_____
_____
_____

cut here

**May we quote your comments in information sheets about the
book or on our website?**

☐ Yes, and you can use my full name.
☐ Yes, but use my initials only and city and state.
☐ Yes, but use "QOD dieter" and city and state
☐ No, please don't quote me in any way

Many thanks!
—John T. Daugirdas, M.D.